A TREATISE ON THE ART OF MIDWIFERY.

SETTING FORTH VARIOUS ABUSES THEREIN, ESPECIALLY AS TO THE PRACTICE WITH INSTRUMENTS

MRS. ELIZABETH NIHELL

Published by Left of Brain Books

Copyright © 2021 Left of Brain Books

ISBN 978-1-396-31841-2

First Edition

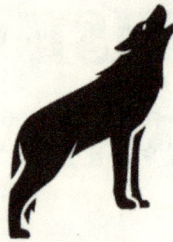

Table of Contents

TO ALL FATHERS, MOTHERS, AND LIKELY SOON TO BE EITHER.

THOUGH the subject of the following sheets is of such universal importance, that it would be difficult to name that human individual, to whom it does not in some measure relate, you, it doubtless, more immediately concerns.

Under no protection then so properly as yours can a work be put, not presumingly calculated to determine your judgment, but only to recommend to you the examination of a point, in which Nature would have such just reproaches to make to you, for cruelty to yourselves, if you was indolently to determine yourselves either without an examination, or on a blind implicit confidence in others; in others, perhaps, interested to mislead you. This last advertence of mine will, more than all that I could offer besides, prove to you my sincere unaffected wish for your favorable acceptance of this essay of mine, on the footing of absolutely no interest but purely yours. And that interest how dear! How sacred! How indispensably ought it to challenge your preference almost to any other interest of your own, and much more surely to any of others.

Happily then for you, in a matter of such common concernment to human-kind, Nature has not been so unjust, nor so unprovident as to place a competent notion of it out of the reach of common sense.

Deign then, for your own sakes, to examine it by that light of Reason, the spring of which is for ever in yourselves. It cannot fail of affording you a sufficient certainty on which to rest your opinion, in a point upon which it is of such deep, such tender importance to you, not to form your resolutions on a wrong one. In virtue of such your own fair examination, the decision will no longer be dangerously and precariously that of others for you, no longer be nothing better than a lightly adopted prejudice, but become truly and meritoriously the genuine result of your own judgment.

But whatever your decision may be, at least to me you can hardly impute it as an offence, my seeking to supply you with matter, whereon to exercise that judgment of yours in so interesting a point. At the worst, I have the consolation of being in my duty, while thus aiming, however deficiently, at providing that with the most tender regard and unfeigned zeal.

I am, respectfully,

Your most devoted, and most faithful humble servant,

ELIZABETH NIHELL.

PREFACE.

THE preservation of so valuable a part of the human Species as pregnant women, as well as that of their dear and tender charge, their children, so powerfully recommended by the voice of Nature and Reason, to all possible human providence for their safe birth, forms an object so sensibly entitled to the private and national care, and even to that of universal society, that all enforcement of its importance would be an injury to the human understanding, or at least to the human heart. It would look too like imagining that it could be wanted.

What I have then to say preliminarily, must chiefly arise from my own due sense of my inequality to the subject of which I presume to treat. Though, if example could be any countenance, I might plead that of so many authors who have, with the utmost confidence and the utmost absurdity, written upon the art of midwifery, without understanding any thing at all of it. The truth is, that my very natural and strong attachment to the profession, which I have long exercised and actually do exercise, created in me an unsuppressible indignation at the errors and pernicious innovations introduced into it, and every day gaining ground, under the protection of Fashion, sillily fostering a preference of men to women in the practice of midwifery: a preference first admitted by credulous Fear, and admitted without examination, upon the so suspicious recommendation of those interested to make that Fear subservient to their selfish ends.

Of these disorders, pernicious as they are to society, I have however been long withheld from taking public notice by far from groundless scruples. Being myself a practitioner, I had just reason to fear, that my representation would have the less influence, from a supposition of personal interest in them. They might naturally enough be construed as the result of a jealousy of profession. I had yet a reason more particular to myself against interfering in this matter. My husband is unhappily for me a surgeon-apothecary: I say unhappily, because though of a business I maintain to be so foreign and distinct from the function which I profess, there might not be wanting, among such as would imagine their private interest attempted at least to be hurt by me, a suspicion that I was indirectly aiming at recommending his advantage in prejudice to theirs. Yet so far, so very far is this from being the case, that the main scope of my essay is to prove, that his business has no relation at all to mine, and that especially as to the particular point I would wish to establish, he is absolutely as indifferent to me as any other person, either of his own profession, or of any other whatsoever. This prejudice then of self-interest being fairly annulled by the appeal to the manifest drift of the work itself, which gives him as formally the exclusion as to any other of his sex, I had still a repugnance to the entering into a discussion of abuses, that could not be laid open without exposing truths, that might have an air of invidiousness or detraction.

Some friends of mine, to whom I communicated my doubts, agreed with me, that there are faults which cannot innocently be revealed, where their manifestation may be attended with some greater evil, but that it could not be right to rank among the faults to be spared any error in an art, where one single false idea, suffered to subsist, may prove the occasion of wounds or torturous death to thousands. On the contrary, the due knowledge of faults of this nature is, in fact, a public benefit. They serve, as one may say, for beacons to the art, they hold a light to it, and show it the rocks it should avoid.

It is certain then, that I have not the least intention to attack any particular persons, any farther than in what I conceive to be false theory, or mispractice in the art I profess; I hope then it will not be imputed to me as unfair or over-presumptuous, if I especially do not over-respect writers or practitioners, who themselves have not respected either common-sense or common-humanity.

Have not some of our modern authors, especially the male-practitioners, who in these later times have treated of midwifery, added new and worse errors of their own to those bequeathed to us by the antients, whom they have insulted, as they themselves will probably one day be, but with more reason, by their successors, if the world should continue blind enough for them to have any in this profession? One would even imagine, that in the criticisms in which they indulge themselves of one another's sistems and instruments, they are inflicting part of the punishment due for their common offences against Nature, in the abuse of an Art, originally intended to assist her. At the same time, even from their own showing, nothing can be plainer, than that their boasted inventions have, under the specious pretence of improvement, fallen from bad to worse, as is ever the case of superstructures on the crazy foundation of false principles.

Read the men-writers on this art, and you will find interspersed in most of them, amidst the most flagrant proofs of their own ignorance of it, reproaches to that of the midwives, too just, perhaps as to some, but shamelessly absurd in them, who to that ignorance substitute their own subtilities of theory, which, when reduced to practice, are infinitely worse than any deficiency in some particular female-practitioners; being mostly, in truth, fit for nothing so much, as to prepare dreadful work for their instruments.

But if they so falsely exalt their own learning above the ignorance of women; they have their reason for it. They seek to drive out of the practice those who stand in the way of their private interest: that private interest, to which the public one is for ever sacrificed under the specious and stale pretext of its advancement.

Can it then be wrong in any of our sex and profession to endeavour, at least, to justify ourselves, and to undeceive the public, of the ill and false impressions which have been given it of our talents and ability? Pernicious prejudices have sometimes their run, like epidemical distempers: and surely it is more for the service of mankind, that their duration should be shortened, than suffered to proceed without at least an endeavour to oppose them.

I should, however, be much more pleased with an exemption from the disagreeable talk of composing the apology of our sex in this matter, it being contrary to that modesty which becomes us so well; but as the men-midwives, in their sistem of exalting their powers of Art over ours of Nature, keep no measures with truth, I see myself forced to do justice to our function, and to manifest the unreasonableness of that contempt, with which they treat and depreciate our services; and with which they have, in favor of their own interest, perhaps too successfully imbued the public.

In this attempt of mine there is no blamable ostentation. If I set in their just light of utility the qualifications of the women of our profession, as to industry, dexterity, ease of execution, patience, constitutional tenderness, and especially natural aptitude, it is no more than practical truth warrants, and the throwing a due light into the matter of comparison requires. Yet I do not wish, that we should pass for any thing beyond what we really are. All the partiality, all the tender feelings it is so natural for me to have for the sufferings of my own sex, would be sufficient to with-hold me from desiring to establish any opinion or practice tending to endanger the personal safety of women in child-birth, or of any thing so dear to them as their children. I am myself a mother.

I own however there are but too few midwives who are sufficiently mistresses in their profession. In this they are some of them but too near upon a level with the men-midwives, with this difference however in favor of the female practitioners, that they are incapable of doing so much actual mischief as the male-ones, oftenest more ignorant than themselves, but who with less tenderness and more rashness go to work with their instruments, where the skill and management of a good midwife would have probably prevented the difficulty, or even after its coming into existence, prove more efficacious towards saving both mother and child; always with due preference however to the mother.

I will also, with the same candor, own that there are some not intirely incapable men-midwives: but they are so very rare, and must for ever necessarily be so, and even, at the best, so inferior to good midwives, that a worse office could scarce be done to mankind, that on so false a supposition as that of a sufficient ability in them, explode the practice of the art by women, because some of them might be exceptionable. And how should it be otherwise, than that some should be more deficient than others? Is there that art in the world, to which the same objection does not lie of different degrees of merit in the professors of it, as well as that of the imperfection of all human arts in general?

In the mean time, the consequences of this unfair conclusion against the women professors of midwifery, in affording the men a plea for supplanting them, do not hitherto appear very advantageous ones to the public. It remains, I fancy, to be proved, that population is any gainer by the diminution of that evil, to which the instruments or other methods of practice, employed by the men, are pretended to be such a remedy.

To examine this point is the object of the following sheets; the work being divided into two parts.

The first treats of our title to the practice of this art, of the pleas used by the men for arrogating to themselves the preference, of the knowledge of Anatomy, of the necessity of the instruments, of the incapacity of women, of the Fashion: and whether the superior safety is on the side of employing men-practitioners.

The answers inserted to each objection, all together, constitute an essay to remove the prejudices, which have been so industriously, and too successfully disseminated against the female practice of this art; and to show that the substitution of the men, more especially of their iron and steel-implements, is attended with greater danger, greater mischiefs, than those which that substitution is pretended to prevent or redress.

The second has more particularly for object to demonstrate the insufficiency, danger, and actual destructiveness of instruments in the art of midwifery. To this purpose I therefore pass all that is needful of them in review, in the several cases, in which the antients and moderns would persuade us they are necessary. I set myself to establish my exceptions to them by uncontestable examples; but above all, by the authority of reason and experience. I take notice of some of the manifest contradictions to be met with in almost all the authors, to one another. I have ventured to subjoin some observations, taken from my own observations and practice, in lieu of what I condemn, and to point out a method of operation, much more plain, more tender, more secure, than the one by instruments. I support this by those general principles, which have happily guided me on all occasions, and from which it is even easy to refute the pretentions and sistem of the instrumentarians, in which I shall note here only three essential defects.

The *first*, in that the origin of the men, insinuating themselves into the practice of midwifery, has absolutely no foundation in the plea of superior safety, and, consequently, can have no right to exact so great a sacrifice as that of decency and modesty.

The *second*, for that they were reduced first to forge the phantom of incapacity in the women, and next the necessity of murderous instruments, as some color for their mercenary intrusion. And, in truth, the faculty of using those instruments is the sole tenure of their usurped office.

The *third*, their disagreement among themselves about, which are the instruments to be preferred; a doubt which, the practices tried upon the lives and limbs of so many women and children trusted to them, have not yet, it seems, resolved, even to this day.

But reserving to treat upon these and other points more at large, in their place, I am to bespeak the reader's candid construction, of my having, especially in the beginning of the first part, transiently availed myself of the authorities of authors, sacred and prophane. It is less that I think truth stands in need of such corroboratives, than to show that it is not destitute of them. It is not by authority, but by reason, that truth, in matters of temporal concernment, claims acceptance from reasonable beings. At the worst, those to whom they may present a tiresome prospect, have but to skip them over; or if they peruse them, they are desired not to forget that no stress is laid on them, beyond their being answers to arguments of the like nature, urged on the opposite side of the question.

Though instruments are not within my sphere of practice; though consequently I have the honor of not being personally very well acquainted with them, nor have I at hand all the original authors who have published their own inventions of them, I have been sufficiently enabled to do justice to their pretentions, by a recourse to those who professedly and fully treat of them. My guide is commonly Monsieur Levret, who is one of the exactest describers of them. Not most certainly that I otherwise prefer him, for of the utility of his forceps I think just as ill as I do of all the rest.

I should have been glad to avoid at once the barren driness of abridgments furnishing no distinct ideas, and the tedious exactness of particularized descriptions and histories; as for example, of the forceps, as well as of errors committed by practitioners; but this medium I could rather wish than hope to keep. I have then been so afraid of obscuring matters by brevity, that of the two I have perhaps run too far into the contrary and less agreeable excess; which, however, in consideration of its favoring explicitness, is not perhaps the most inexcusable one.

I wish I could make an apology as receivable by reader, who will doubtless be justly disgusted at the repetitions I have too little scrupled the making of the same thoughts, and even sometimes of the same expressions. Yet I dare bespeak, from his candor, some indulgence to the confession of a fault, it will easily be perceived I could not well escape, without the worse inconvenience to himself, of his being perplexed with references back to past pages, besides, that sometimes a chain of argument would be broke, consequently weakened, by the suppression of some link of it, on account of the matter having been elsewhere already employed in other connexions.

Upon the whole, I throw myself, with the more confidence, on the favorable acceptance of the public, from my consciousness of its not being but with the best intentions for the good of society that I hazard this production: and have therefore reason to hope, that it will occasionally be remembered, that my object is purely that of representing a truth, and not of recommending a composition.

PART THE FIRST.

WHOEVER considers the absolute necessity of the art of midwifery, will readily allow it a place among the capital ones in the primeval times of the world. All the other arts are no further necessary to man, than to procure him the conveniencies or luxuries of life; that of midwifery is of indispensable necessity to his living at all, imploring as he does its aid for his introduction into life. Without this art the earth itself must soon become dispeopled and a desert, whereas by means of it men have been multiplied, with inconceivable rapidity.

In conformity to its claim importance, this art appeared in all its lustre among the Jews, the Egyptians, the Athenians and Romans, and indeed in all nations during thousands of ages. Nor was the confinement of the exercise of it to women deemed any derogation to it. It even gave honor to its professors of that sex. Socrates, so ennobled by his character of being the greatest philosopher in all antiquity, did not disdain to boast himself the son of a very able midwife Phanarete, as may be seen in Plato's book on science, in Diogenes Laertius and others.

Among the Egyptians and the Greeks it cannot be hard to conceive what emulation, what ardor it must have excited among the women of that profession, the custom of distributing prizes to those of the greatest merit in it, in the face of the people. No one is ignorant of the power of honors and distinction to bring arts to perfection.

But from the instant the midwives sunk into dis-esteem, and whatever that has happened, it will be found by woeful experience, that only the art itself has suffered in the very midst of the most falsely boasted improvements, but that human-kind itself has much and very justly to complain of the change.

The native inconstancy and levity of the French nation opened the first inlet, in these modern-times, to men-practitioners. In antient history we meet with but one feeble attempt of that sort, which however soon gave way to the united powers of modesty and common sense. In France, and may it not be same case soon here! the women of a competent class of life and education, begin to decline forming themselves for this profession, as beneath them, considering the slight put upon those women who exercise it.

Nor has this injustice remained unpunished. Many women have found, by severe experience, their having been enemies to themselves, in abandoning or slighting those of their own sex, from whom, at their greatest need, they used to receive the most effectual service, and who alone are capable of discharging their duty by them, with that sympathy for their pains, that tender affectionate concern, which may so naturally be expected from those who have been, are, or may be subject to the same infirmities.

Many out of a distrust inspired them of midwives, have thrown themselves into the hands of men, who have promised them infinitely more than they were able to perform; and who behind all the tender alluring words, of superior skill and safety in the employing of them, conceal the ideas with which they are full, of cutting, hacking, plucking out piece-meal, or tearing limb from limb.

The murder of so many children, the fruits of their bowels, might, one would imagine, have induced mothers to consider this point a little more carefully. Yet, through the prevalence of groundless fears, and of imaginary dangers they have run into real ones, and have sometimes found their death precisely where they sought their life; and not seldom where nature has even favored them enough in their labor, for them not to need any extraordinary ministry of art, the men have put them to cruel and dangerous tortures.

Notwithstanding some examples, and many violent presumptions of such mal-treatment, too many women have been so miserably misled by fashion, as to prefer the betraying the cause of their own sex, and the subjecting themselves to those who deceive them with false hopes, to the entrusting their preservation to those of their own sex, in the hands of which the care of it has been for so many ages, with so much reason, and such little cause of complaint.

Yet we do not see that any of these men-midwifes have been capable of forming a good midwife. On the contrary, we see, that in order to remedy the abuses, or rather to prevent the fatal accidents which every day occur in the practice of a profession so necessary to the preservation of the human species, they were in France obliged to have recourse to one of the ablest midwives in that kingdom, who was placed at the head of the practice in the Hôtel Dieu at

Paris, to preside over the lyings-in there, and to found and cultivate that inexhaustible seminary of excellent female practitioners, who have actually restored the art to its antient degree of esteem, with all fair judges. These worthy proficients have been so public-spirited, as to communicate their talents and knowledge to a number of surgeons, who never had any reason to be ashamed of the lessons they assiduously took from the midwives, unless indeed for themselves not being able to come up to them in the practice, so true it is, that the business is not at all natural to them.

Yet have even many of those very men-practitioners, influenced by that self-interest which has such a power in all human affairs, revolted against their mistresses in the art, and their benefactresses. They have, at various times, commenced lawsuits, about the Hôtel Dieu at Paris, in order to get the lyings-in there committed to them: but the administrators, the persons of a just sense of things, together with the parliament of that town, ever attentive to decency, without excluding the due regard to the preservation of the subjects, have constantly opposed and frustrated the pretentions of these innovators. These again thus disappointed, were forced to content themselves with practicing upon some women of quality, under the favor and protection of some of the old ladies of the court of Lewis XIV. who had their reasons for propagating this fashion. And now these innovators, not without a due proportion of ingratitude to the injustice, began to run down the midwives, and exalt themselves. The novelty prevailed, and the contagion of example soon communicated itself to the provinces, and thence into neighbouring nations. A few men perhaps of real abilities, but governed by the most sordid interest, associated to their party a number of the most ignorant and unexpert practitioners, but who served to fill up the cry, and made a common cause against the midwives, whose pretended insufficiency was now to be pleaded in favor of themselves being admitted to supplant them. Nor was the concurrent attestation in their favor, of so many ages, during which the practice was entirely in female hands, to weigh any thing against the boasts of their own superior ability. They picked up and sounded loud a few real instances perhaps, and undoubtedly many false ones of faults of practice in women: though were the numbers of human creatures, who have barbarously perished by the unskilfulness of the practitioners, to be fairly liquidated, it would appear that fewer have been the victims of female ignorance, than of the presumption and indexterity of the men. The women are undoubtedly liable to error: there have even been monsters of iniquity among them, but certainly in no number to form a general prejudice against them: but as to the men they are all of them, as will be more fully demonstrated hereafter, naturally incapable of the exercise of this profession. A history of their murders might even be collected out of the books written by them to establish their superiority over the women. From Deventer, Mauriceau, and the most celebrated of their writers, amongst many excellent observations in the way of the chirurgical art, many of the grossest absurdities have escaped, where they transgress its bounds and go into that of midwifery. Some of those absurdities too are so glaring, that they have not even been overlooked by themselves.

Many persons in Holland, having set up for men-midwives, without being duly qualified, the government thought proper to interfere, and consequently there was an ordinance issued on the 31st of January, 1747, by which it was enjoined, that no one should practice in the quality of man-midwife, or exercise this art, unless he were especially authorized for this function, by a certificate of his having undergone a sufficient examination before capable and intelligent judges for that purpose appointed.

It will appear, in the sequel of this work, that it were to be wished, for the sake of the good that would redound from it, to the preservation of the human species, both in parent and child, that those who are entrusted with the public welfare, would establish the same regulation in the British dominions, to expel and exclude from the art all the ignorant pretenders of either sex, who are, in fact worse than the Herods of society. The cruelty of Herod extended to no more than to the infants; not to the mothers; that of such pretenders to both.

If their conduct was to be examined with attention, how many fatal mistakes would be discovered in the practitioners of both sexes? But I dare aver it more in the men than in the women-practitioners. With what horror would not there in these be remarked, tearings, rendings, and tortures of no use to which they put both the mother and the child? One, upon some most learnedly erroneous hypothesis, pulls and hauls the arm of an innocent infant yet living, so that he plucks it off; or repels it with such violence, that he breaks it: another unmercifully opens the infant's head, and takes the brain out: some bring the whole away piece-meal: operations often to be defended only by hard words and harder hearts.

13

Nor need this procedure astonish. Every thing is at the disposal, I had almost said, at the mercy of these executioners: but have they any? All their handy-work is transacted in private, and remains buried in the tomb of oblivion. The parents suspecting nothing, think every thing has been done, according to art, that is to say, very right. The operator thinks he has done nothing but his duty, and is highly satisfied with himself, after he has ordered some draughts for his patient. The magistrate knows no injury done to the subject, or is insensible to the consequences from the same spirit of confidence. In the mean time, a husband loses a fine child, or a beloved wife, perhaps both; children, a tender mother, and if they are of the same sex, have the same fate to dread for themselves. The man-midwife is clear, for only saying, that he has done all for the best. But this is probably true too, as to the intention; but as to the fact, it shall be shewn that there is often great reason to doubt it.

Be this observed, without offence to the few able men-midwives who are masters enough of the business, not to deserve the reproaches due to by much the greater number of rash and ignorant pretenders to it: whose practice, well examined, would bring to light such terrible truths, as would alarm even the legislature to provide a remedy against the danger.

In contradiction to this, it may be urged, that the practice by women is susceptible upon that account, of superior objections. That remains now to be examined. The chief object of this work being a fair discussion, which of the two sexes is the most appropriated by nature and art, to the exercise of this function.

To this end, I shall present, in a candid view, the two opinions which, on this point, divide the English yet more than they do the French. Most of the surgeons, all the men-midwives, no doubt, many apothecaries, a number of women and nurses maintain, that midwifery is the business of the men: whilst on the other hand, the best part of the able physicians, with many other persons of both sexes, defend the contrary side of the question, and insist on this art being, for many invincible reasons, solely the province of female practitioners.

Not to lose sight of the fundamental arguments and proofs brought to support respectively these two opinions, I shall place them in parallel with one another, in form of objections and answers. The objections made to women-practitioners precede the answers. If the men-midwives, or their partizans, shall think I have omitted any thing that makes for them, or against us, or have any stronger or more essential arguments to oppose, I shall endeavour to satisfy them.

OBJECTION THE FIRST.

Regard ought to be paid to prior possession. The art of midwifery being a branch of the art of physic, must have been originally in the hands of man, the inventor of all arts.

ANSWER.

The just deference so universally paid to holy writ will, I presume, allow no prejudice to be found against my availing myself of those inferences and decisions to be drawn from it, which are so agreeable to the eternal laws of common sense.

If the arts and sciences, acquired by experience, and by acts often repeated, had, as they certainly were not invented by men only, that could not at least be said of those acts of the human life, which are indispensably necessary to its preservation. Such faculties may with more propriety be termed instinctive, than invented ones. The faculties of eating, of drinking, of lying down to rest, common to both sexes, are not perhaps more natural, more matter of instinct, than the faculty of one woman assisting another in her labor-pains being appropriated to the female sex.

There is no occasion to give one's imagination the torture to account for Eve's delivering herself or her first children. There is no reason to establish it as an absolute necessity that Adam should have assisted Eve in her first lyings-in; whose labor-pains might not only be less severe, than they afterwards became in accomplishment for the curse pronounced on the human race for the sin of those first parents, but also more consonant to piety, to believe that God, being the best of fathers, infused into Eve knowledge sufficient of the manner of delivering herself; a manner more natural and more conformable to the ideas of that decency imprinted with has own hand in the human heart, in no point more strongly, nor more universally, than in this matter of the

15

woman lying-in, when both men and women have an equal repugnance to the interposition of any assistance, but that of the female sex, to which the faculty of ministering in that case seems innate.

But admitting even that Adam, for the want of females for that function, before the daughters of Eve were grown up to a capacity of it, actually did assist Eve, in the seasons of her delivery; that would establish no inference of right for the future: since we know that their children and descendants in time following did not make use of men to lay the women.

In Genesis, chap. xxxv. ver. 17, there is mention made of Rachel's midwife. In the same book, chap. xxxviii. ver. 27, and 28. we see they were intelligent midwives. Thamar being with child. "It came to pass in the time of her travail, that behold, twins were in her womb."

Ver. 28. "And it came to pass that when she travailed, that the one put out his hand, and the *Midwife* took and bound upon his hand a scarlet thread, saying, this came out first."

And here I intreat the reader not to impute to me an idea so absurd as that of meaning to defend an erroneous practice solely from the antiquity of it; I intend nothing further by this citation, than to prove the antiquity itself, which if not decisive in favor of the practice by women, can at least be no prejudice against it.

OBJECTION THE SECOND.

The art of midwifery being equally noble for its subject as for its end, since it is the only one which enjoys the prerogative of saving, at one operation of the hand, more than one individual at once; ought the less noble sex to dispute pre-eminence in it with the men? On tracing things back to the remotest distance of times, it must be allowed, that if the women, through a mistaken modesty, in those times of ignorance and simplicity, commonly made use of midwives, it may be presumed there were also men-practitioners employed in difficult cases.

ANSWER.

Readily granting that the art is a noble one; noble in its subject and ends: all that I am surprised at is, that the men did not find it out sooner. Probably the nobility of this art is only begun to be sounded so high by the men, till they discovered the possibility of making it a lucrative one to themselves. Then indeed the ignorance and incapacity of the poor women for it, came all of a sudden to be doubted and despised. The art with all its nobility was for so many ages thought beneath the exercise of the noble sex: it was held unmanly, indecent, and they might safely have added impracticable for them. But had even any of the medical profession not thought so, there is great reason to think the rest of mankind would have viewed their interested endeavors to usurp this province from the female sex, in the light they deserve. It was only for the eternal fondness which prevails among the French for novelties, that paved the way for the admission of so dangerous and indecent an one, as that of mens making a common practice of midwifery, and taking it out of the womens hands, to which it was so much more natural.

I am here far from wishing to enter into a contest with the men, on the superiority and excellence they assume over the women; though not quite so indisputable perhaps as is commonly imagined. All that I contend for, to the purpose of the present question, is, that there are certain employments and vocations, which are generally and naturally more proper for one sex than for another. A woman would seem to aim at something above her sex, that would set up an academy for teaching to fence, or ride the great horse. But a man sinks beneath his sex, who interferes in the female province. It is not with quite so good a grace as a woman that he would spin, make beds, pickle and preserve, or officiate as a midwife. Be this observed without impeachment of the superiority of men.

Open books, sacred and profane, you will find that the Egyptians were not so simple as Dr. Smellie would give us to understand they were; when in the beginning of his introduction, pages 1st and 2d, he grants us, out of his special grace and favor, "that in the first ages the practice of the art of midwifery was *altogether* in the hands of women, and that men were never employed but in the utmost extremity: indeed (says he) it is natural to suppose, that while the *simplicity* of the early ages remained, women would have recourse to none but persons of their own sex, in diseases *peculiar* to it: accordingly we find that in Egypt midwifery was practiced by women."

According to scripture, however, the sorcerers of Egypt were not so very simple neither, since they had art enough to imitate some of the miracles of

Moses, in transforming their rods into serpents, water into blood, and covering the land with frogs.[1] All this did not favor of simplicity.

The Egyptians[2] have ever passed for the most intelligent and enlightened of all the other nations of the earth, who respected them as oracles of wisdom and found philosophy. They are the first people who established systematically rules of good government. This profound and serious nation saw early the true end of human policy; and virtue being the principal foundation and cement of all society, they industriously cultivated it. At the head of all virtues they placed that of gratitude. The honor attributed to them of being the most grateful of men, shews that they were also the most social. They had an inventive genius: their Mercuries, who filled Egypt with surprising discoveries, scarce left any thing wanting to the perfection of their understanding, or to the convenience and happiness of life. The first people among whom libraries were known to exist, is that of Egypt. In short, so far from being simple or ignorant, they excelled in all the sciences. There were indeed among them no *men-midwives*; but to make up for this deficiency, they had, it seems, excellent midwives.

Besides it is even ridiculous to confine the practice of midwifery by females only to early ages. Who does not know, that it was so in all ages, and in all countries, till just the present one, in which the innovation has crept into something of a fashion into two or three countries. The exceptions before, or any where else, to the general rule, are so few, that they are scarce worth mentioning.

But to return to the so *simple* Egyptians. We read in Exodus, chap. i. v. 15. and following, that Pharaoh said to the midwives, "When ye do the office of midwife to the Hebrew women, and set them upon the stools, if it be a son then ye shall kill him, but if it be a daughter she shall live.

17. But the midwives feared God, and did not as the king of Egypt commanded them, but saved the men-children alive."

The king reproached them, as may be seen in the same place.

Why did not Pharaoh give the same order to the men-midwives, if there had been any such employed in difficult or extraordinary pains? (as Mr. Smellie supposes.) Or rather, if the king had not thought it too unnatural

---

[1] Exod. Chap. vii. and viii.
[2] Diod. Sic. Herodotus.

for women to be delivered by men, he certainly would not have failed to have commanded it, especially on perceiving that the midwives had deceived him. This would have been a fine occasion to have forbidden them their function, and for the men-practitioners to have come into vogue. The men would certainly have been of the two not the improperest to have executed the intentions of the tyrant: as tender-heartedness is surely not more the character of their sex, than of the women. Besides, their instruments would have served admirably to have thinned the species, without distinction of the sexes. They might also have concealed the barbarity of the murders by such instruments, under the pretext of their necessity from hard-labors, as the midwives excused their disobedience under that of easy ones, which had rendered their aid superfluous.

OBJECTION THE THIRD.

So many authors as have wrote on the art of midwifery, from the age in which Hippocrates flourished, whom we look on as the first and father of the men-midwives, with the disciples whom he formed, and their successors, do not they satisfactorily prove the antiquity of man-midwives?

ANSWER.

As for satisfactorily, no. It can only be concluded from this objection, that the ignorance of the pretended men-midwives is very antient; and yet posterior by much to the function of the midwives, since that is coeval with the world itself, embraces all times, extends through all parts of the earth, whereas we hear nothing of the other till the times of Hippocrates.

Nevertheless I greatly respect Hippocrates, and all the authors who have treated of this art. Some thanks are due to them, though but from those whom they have set to work in our days. Consider but the most celebrated authors among them down to our times, there may be found in them great progresses by degrees, especially in our modern writers on this subject. Yet the most intelligent of them feel and confess that the matter is yet far from exhausted. For after having studied all the treatises we have upon it, there may, there must be perceived an aberration and emptiness with which the understanding remains unsatisfied, and feels that much is yet wanting to the requisite perfection.

Notwithstanding likewise the veneration confessedly due to Hippocrates, I cannot dispense myself from saying the truth, he might be and doubtless was an excellent physician: he has wrote upon all the female disorders, and on the means of delivering them; he may have been consulted in his time, but he can never pass for an able man-midwife. His writings contain some violent remedies and strange prescriptions for women in labor, which must be the produce of the most dangerous ignorance of what is proper for them in that condition.

This author was also evidently ignorant of what concerns preternatural deliveries, as indeed were his successors till the beginning of the last century.

To prove what I advance, there needs no recourse back to very remote times: it will be sufficient to peruse the treatises of Ambrose Paræus, Jacques Guillimeau, Peter-Paul Bienassis, printed 1602, and even that of De la Motte, who is of this century, to own, that the practice of the men-midwives was far from having attained any degree of perfection.

The manner in which the antients proceeded, when the child presented in an untoward situation, is a fully convincing proof thereof; since they obstinately, in such cases, continued their efforts to reduce it to its natural situation, in spite of a thousand difficulties and dangers, instead of bringing it away footling, as is now done by all who understand the right practice.

Hippocrates is the first who discovered that wonderful secret of killing the child, and bringing it away piece-meal from the mother's womb. He advises it, in the manner taken notice of by Dr. Smellie, in his introduction, (page 10. & seq.) I do not know whether it is from that branch of practice that he adopts him for "the father of midwifery" (p. 4.) but, what is certain is, that Galen, and all the successors of Hippocrates, till towards the end of the last century, exactly followed his method of not delivering women in hard labors, but by the means of murderous instruments. I shall not here detain myself with rehearsing the long legend Mr. Smellie gives us of all the authors who have written on this subject to the time of Ambrose Paræus; time when to the progresses made by the midwives of the Hôtel Dieu at Paris in the art of midwifery, it was owing, that the surgeons, guided by the superior lights, made some greater progresses towards perfection.

That the reader however may not suspect me of exaggeration, or over-training points, I request of him to suspend his judgment, to have the patience to hear me out to the end, and he will find, that I have here advanced nothing but what in the sequel stands clearly and manifestly proved.

OBJECTION THE FOURTH.

In a word, the manual operation of midwifery is an art, a science, and as such consequently more competently to be professed by men, than by women. It is making the art cheap, say the moderns, to allow the practice of it to women.

ANSWER.

I agree with you in the first part of your objection: but I absolutely deny the consequences.

There are women, who, besides the gifts received from nature, and improved by study, by reading, and experience, who succeed much more easily than men in the practice. To say the truth, nature has, in this point, been even lavish to the women, for this art is a gift innate to them.

I will however own, that not all women indistinctly are proper for this business; that there must be natural dispositions cultivated by art; that a purely speculative knowledge is not sufficient; that there are required good intellects, memory, strength of body and mind, sentiments, some taste, and practiced joined to theory; so that when I say that the women are born with dispositions for this art; this can only be understood in general, and relatively to the men, among whom those dispositions are more rare, because they are less natural to them in this branch.

Would it not be a sort of blasphemy against the divine providence to maintain, that what God has placed and left in possession of the women, was fitter for the men? the attentive, beneficent, and tender manner with which he governed his people elect, obliges us to believe that he omitted nothing of what was necessary or advantageous to it, since he regarded that people as his own particular dominion and appendage; honoring it with his presence, like a master in his dwelling-house, or a father in his family. He had taken pleasure in the forming and instructing it from it's infancy. He put the women in possession of the art of midwifery, he blessed, approved, and recompenced the midwives. It is but just, that men should hear and keep silence where God speaks. They may think themselves happy, to learn from him the true secrets of nature, and not from those pretended doctors who abandon the rules of truth to cleave to themselves; who, instead of her, present us with a phantom of their own creation, who, in short, would make us the worshippers of their dreams and imaginations.

The women have for them the authority of God, who has declared himself in their favor; they have for them the authority of men from one pole to the other, who have in all ages made use of the female ministry in this art. Such a plurality of votes has surely some claim to prevalence, especially, since it is founded upon the natural order of things, upon truth and reason supported by experience. This experience we have on our side: none can deny it, without denying self-evidence.

One would think there is a kind of curse attends the operations of men-practitioners, as I dare aver it for a truth, that difficult and fatal labors have never been so rise, or so frequent, as since the intermeddling of the men. Whereas, God has ever so blessed the work of the midwives, that never were lyings-in so happily conducted, nor so successful, as when the practice was entirely in their hands.

Open the book of Numbers, you will observe, that God having ordered Moses to number his people: out of seventy individuals of the family of Jacob, who had come to dwell in Egypt, two hundred and forty years before, there had issued above six hundred thousand men fit to carry arms, without taking into the account an almost infinite multitude of children, of youths under twenty years of age, of women, of old men, besides a whole tribe, that of Levi, which was entirely set apart for the divine worship.

OBJECTION THE FIFTH.

There is no such thing as being a good practitioner of midwifery without understanding anatomy: now this science is the province of a man, of a physician, or surgeon, not of a woman.

ANSWER.

It is sufficient that a woman understands and knows the structure and mechanical disposition of the internal parts which more particularly distinguish her sex; that she can discern the container from the contents, what belongs to the mother what belongs to the child, as well as what is foreign to both. In short, she ought to be skilled enough to give full satisfaction to all questions that the most able anatomist could put to her, in respect to that part purely necessary to the art of midwifery, and to its operations with mastery and safety.

Now the midwife, especially one instructed in hospitals, ought to be well acquainted with all that is essential and necessary to that effect; and she cannot but be so, unless she is of herself incapable, or that those who are charged with the instruction of pupils, wrong the confidence of the public.

I myself know more than one midwife, so well educated as to be able to give demonstrations on this subject, to analize things by their names, either upon drawings of them, upon skeletons, or upon the originals themselves. It is true, that these poor midwives do not understand anatomy enough to make dissections; but I fancy that the ladies who want assistance in their lyings-in; are not very curious of having one that can dissect instead of delivering them.

Prophane history has preserved to us the names and talents of a number of illustrious women who have distinguished themselves in all kinds of arts. Cleopatra queen of Egypt, is one of the first ladies that have written on the art of midwifery. Mr. Smellie, in his introduction, endeavours to render doubtful this quality of queen and princess, with a design, probably to weaken the credit of it, or rather out of contempt to the women; but as all those who have made collections of antient history, assure us, that notwithstanding the wars in which this princess was engaged, she did not neglect an assiduous application to physic, I had rather adhere to their authority, than to that of Mr. Smellie.

In Greece, Aspasia, and a number of other celebrated women, quoted by various authors, have applied themselves to our profession, and have left behind them valuable works on the method of delivering women, and of managing them both before and after their lying-in.

Madam Justin, midwife to the Electress of Brandenbourg, has also given us a very good treatise. Several professed midwives appointed to form the

23

apprentices of the Hôtel Dieu at Paris, have written very clearly on the same subject, without however being mistresses of any more anatomy, than what was sufficient for their business.

OBJECTION THE SIXTH.

The different instruments which the men have invented in aid of, and supplement to the deficiency of nature, and of which they are frequently obliged to make use in different labors, ought not to be put into the hands of midwives: and were it but for this reason alone, they ought to be excluded from the practice of this art. As, why multiply attendants unnecessarily? A man-midwife, with his instruments which he ought always to have about him, is enough for every thing: whereas a midwife, if the case requires instruments, will be obliged to have recourse to a man: consequently double embarrassment; double expence.

ANSWER.

The keen instrumentarians bring an argument they imagine capable of banishing or exterminating all the midwives. The men, they say, enjoy alone the glorious privilege of using instruments, in order, as they pretend, to assist nature. But let them, I intreat of them, answer, whether if the question could be decided by votes, where is the kingdom, where is the nation, where is the town, where, in short, is the person that would prefer iron and steel to a hand of flesh, tender, soft, duly supple, dextrous, and trusting to its own feelings for what it is about: a hand that has no need of recourse to such an extremity as the use of instruments, always blind, dangerous, and especially for ever useless?

What has engaged men to invent and bequeath to their successors so many wonderful productions, for such they imagine them? Is it not the thirst of fame and money? These gentry have judged, that they ought to spare no lucubrations, no labor of the head, no efforts of the tongue and pen to procure themselves a strange reputation, supported by these horrible instruments. But these lucubrations, this labor of the head, would have been much better employed in seeking for the means of absolutely doing without them, as our good female practitioners have ever done, and as those of them still do, who are instructed in the right practice.

We are no longer in the times of the Pharaohs and the Herods, who mercilessly massacred the innocents; we are no longer in the times of those pure Arabs, who were the inventors of a number of cruel operations, and of several instruments, which often cause more apprehension and terror to a woman in labor, though concealed from her sight, but never from her imagination, than the actual presence of all the apparatus of the rack, where that torture is in use.

It were to be wished, that all the men-midwives, who had wrote on this matter, had suppressed the mention of their instruments; for as their books often fall into the hands of women, so deeply interested as the sex is in that subject, it is not to be imagined what bad effects they have. Their variations among themselves would be sufficient to frighten the women: you meet with authors condemning in the morning the over-night's sentiment. I can observe them losing their way in systematical errors, which explain nothing to me, and in which nothing can be discovered but disagreement with one another, and with themselves. The wisest and most able of them, after having well examined all the kinds of instruments hitherto invented, have doubtless seen and been convinced of their ridiculousness and usefulness, but all of them have not hitherto dared to speak out and say as much.

The most interested of them would fain persuade us, that, in their display of a whole armory of instruments, they have discovered the philosopher's stone of midwifery, in virtue of which they have a right to wrest out of the women's hands, the practice of an art, which nature has appropriated them. But certainly the point, and the whole point is, to find an expert dexterous hand, the sex is out of the question, provided the work is done to the satisfaction of society, it seems to me that nothing more need be required.

Objection the Seventh.

It is only for the ignorant to be so rash as to raise an out-cry against the use of all instruments; people who do not know the absolute necessity there is for employing them on certain occasions. This clamor must proceed "from the interested views of some low, obscure and illiterate practitioners, both male

25

and female, who think that they find their account in decrying the practice of their neighbours." Such is the objection in the words of Dr. Smellie, in his Treatise on Midwifery (page 241.) and for this panegyric, he prepares us in his Introduction (page 55.) where, speaking of the midwives of Hôtel Dieu of Paris, he first indeed tells us, that the surgeons had, in that hospital, perfected themselves in the art of midwifery; but then for fear that from thence occasion might be taken of saying, that to women it was they were beholden for that perfection; he takes care immediately after to add, that what "got the better of those ridiculous prejudices which the fair sex had used to entertain," was, that the women or midwives of this hospital "had recourse to the assistance of men in all difficult cases of midwifery."

ANSWER.

These gentlemen will permit me to tell them that they make great pretentions, and prove little or rather nothing. Calling hard names with a disdainful tone, and with airs of triumph, are not overwhelming reasons.

But to the point. Those who reject instruments, say you, do not know what they are: they reject them from ignorance. This is soon said. Nevertheless a number of authors, much more experienced and versed in the matter than Dr. Smellie, are of this opinion. Deventer exclaims against instruments; Viardel does the same; Levret admits none but those of his own invention, and rejects universally all others; and well might he except his own, since he wrote only to recommend them. Delamotte was not very fond of instruments: he tells us in his preface, that in a course of thirty years practice, he had not twice made use of the crotchet, though he had an extent of country forty leagues round, in which he regularly exercised his profession, insomuch as to have four lyings-in in a day under his management.

I have very exactly read almost all the modern authors who have written on this art; and have been surprized to observe that whilst, on one hand, they agree, they own, that in England, France, and Holland, people are much come off, or undeceived, as to all those dangerous or mortal instruments of which the antients made use, such as the short broad-bladed knife, (call it, if you please, a pen-knife) the bistory, the crotchets, &c. especially since the invention of the new forceps, or tire-tête: on the other hand, these same doctors tell you, that recourse must be had to crotchets, or to the Cæsarean operation, when the new forceps will not do. A comfortable resource this, in an instrument so boasted as the best discovery that has been made since the creation of the world, and for which we are indebted to the moderns!

I have also scrupulously examined all that authors have been pleased to say of great, wonderful and magnificent, with regard to the new forceps of Palfin, as it now stands after infinite corrections, as well in foreign countries, as in this one, which have dignified it with the name of English forceps; and I find all these great elogiums reduced, at the most, to no more than the proving, as clear as the fun, that is allowable for an operator, extremely able and extremely prudent, to make use of it, when the business might be perfectly well done without it.

From thence I deduce my demonstration directly opposite to the pretentions of Dr. Smellie and of his followers. According to the instrumentarians, and according to certain doctors, there are certain occasions, certain cases, in which there is an absolute necessity for employing the forceps. If we will hearken to and follow other doctors of more celebrity and credit, it is not right to make use of it, but when one may very well do without it: for example, after the having obviated all the obstacles which retard the delivery, after having, with the hands only, dis-engaged the head or the shoulders of the child, without which (say these same writers) the instrument would be found insufficient or useless; this palpably implies the being able to do without it. Now since it is not allowable, in good practice, to make use of it, but when it is perfectly needless to use it at all, there is then no absolute necessity for it; as surely, what can be done without, is not absolutely necessary. Be this only transiently remarked. For I reserve most convincingly to prove this proposition in the second part of this work. There I shall treat of all the instruments of our antients and our moderns, and besides an enumeration of them shall demonstrate their danger and uselessness. In the mean time, it must be owned, that either Mr. Smellie has been much mis-informed of what passes at the Hôtel Dieu of Paris, in the ward of the lying-in women, or else, which I the least believe, is not sincere in the account he gives us, that the women of that hospital "had recourse to the assistance of men, in all the difficult cases of midwifery;" which, he observes, "got the better of those ridiculous prejudices the fair sex had been used to entertain." That is to say, in preference of midwives to men-practitioners.

I frequented this Hôtel Dieu two whole years, before being received an apprentice-midwife, which I accomplished with great difficulty, on account of being born a subject of England, and consequently a foreigner there: my admission, however, I gained at length, through the favor, protection, and special recommendation of his royal highness the duke of Orleans. Now, I dare aver, that in all the time before, and after I was admitted there, I never but once saw Mr. Boudou, surgeon-major called, who did nothing more than to make us, one after another, *touch* the patient, about whom we had been embarrassed; and as he interrogated, he made us discover an *uterus* full of schirrous callosities, which joined to its obliquities, impeded the palpation of it properly with the hand, the orifice being very difficult to come at. Every thing, however, was done without his help, and very successfully. And most certainly we should have spared him the trouble of coming at all into our ward, if the head-midwife, who was a little capricious in her temper, had not taken it into her head to keep us in our perplexity, which engaged us to send for Mr. Boudou without her knowledge, and for which she was afterwards heartily angry with us.

I never once saw an occasion in which there was any necessity for using instruments, though in my time we had, at least, five or six hundred women a month to deliver.

Very far then are the midwives from having often occasion of recourse to the assistance of the men, in difficult cases; and indeed to those prejudiced in favor of men-practitioners, it may, though true, appear strange, that in a place where there are every year so many thousand women delivered, and consequently many difficult labors amongst them, and even cases of monsters, there is no recourse to the surgeon-major but in the last occurrence, which falls out very rarely.

About eighteen or twenty years ago, Madam Poor, head-midwife of this hospital, delivered a woman of a monster with two heads, with no help but only her fingers and a young prentice. Not an instrument was employed: no man assisted her. The child was christened, and died presently after. The mother remained some months upon recovery, and did perfectly well. This fact requires no proofs, being of such public notoriety. The monster was carried to St. Cosmo's, where any surgeon may see it. I served my time with this same mistress some years after this kind of prodigy had happened.

As to what I have advanced concerning the procedure in the wards of the lying-in women, should my testimony appear in the least suspicious, I appeal to the justice and veracity of all the doctors in England, who have been at the Hôtel Dieu at Paris, who cannot but confirm what I have said. In the mean time Mr. De la Motte, who passes for an author of credit may certify, the same. Here follows what he says in his preface to his observations, page 2.

"One would think (says this author) from reading the books of Messieurs Mauriceau and Peu, that it was impossible to succeed in the practice of midwifery, without having operated at Paris in the lying-in ward of the Hôtel Dieu. It is true, that this hospital is the best school in Europe; and that I would have ardently wished to have been admitted to the operations of midwifery during the five years I staid in that hospital: but as there is no more than *one* surgeon *only*, who is in charge to attend when he is called to consultation with the midwives, and that it is a place which goes only by favor, I was force to content myself with following in quality of topical surgeon, to the physicians who performed their visits there. So that I followed only, for six months, three physicians in their rounds there, during which time I applied myself to examine the conduct observed by those gentlemen, to preserve the women after their lying-in from the accidents which follow thereon. By this means I made myself amends for my want of recommendation; but I can safely say, that during the six months I was admitted in the above-mentioned quality, there was no more than one extraordinary labor, which was that of a child engaged in the passage, where the presence of a surgeon was required, and which however was terminated without any other help than that of patience. And yet there were (so far back as then) from three hundred and fifty, to four hundred pregnant women, who were all delivered by the apprentices, and rarely by the Dame De la Marche, at that time, head midwife of the hospital: so I am persuaded, that those who boast of having lain a great many women there, exaggerate furiously."

For me, I dare yet to go farther, and will maintain it, that those persons impose upon the public in such boasts: since the naturalized surgeons, those of the nation, those of Paris itself, have no right to come into our ward. There is no one admitted but the surgeon-major, whose place is a place of favor, and rather matter of form than any thing else. Much more then are strangers excluded, and the truth is, that they never did, nor ever do operate there.

As to reproach which Mr. Smellie makes to us of being interested, I can, for myself, prove that I have delivered gratuitously, and in pure charity above nine hundred women. I doubt much, whether our critic can say as much, unless he reckons it for a charity, that which he exercised on his automaton or machine, which served him for a model of instruction to his pupils. This was a wooden statue, representing a woman with child, whose belly was of leather, in which a bladder full, perhaps, of small beer, represented the uterus. The bladder was stopped with a cork, to which was fastened a string of packthread to tap it, occasionally, and demonstrate in a palpable manner the flowing of the red-colored waters. In short, in the middle of the bladder was a wax-doll, to which were given various positions.

By this admirably ingenious piece of machinery, were formed and started up an innumerable and formidable swarm of men-midwives, spread over the town and country. By his own confession, he has made in less than ten years nine hundred pupils, without taking into the account the number of midwives whom he has trained up, and formed in so miraculous a manner. See the preface of this author. He speaks of his *machine* in the first page, and p.5, of the number of his pupils.

Now as to theses worthy pupils, must not they be finely enabled to judge of the situation of women with child, and of that of their fœtus? Must not they be deeply skilled in that branch of anatomy? Must not they acquire a habit of the touch exquisitely nice, exquisitely just, for discerning the proportion and analogy between a mere wooden machine, and a body, sensible, delicate, animated, and well organized?

I hope too that it is an injustice done to that doctor, by those who say that his pupils have too often a way of hurrying out of the waters, which can only serve to render the labor more dry, consequently more laborious, and by that means furnish a handle for setting their instruments to work. If this should be so, as once more I hope it is not, may not the bad habit they will have contracted during their pupilship, of drawing the small-beer out of their wooden-woman, have contributed to this method of practice?

In the mean time, does it become a doctor to call us interested, who himself, for three guineas in nine lessons, made you a man-midwife, or a female one, by means of this most curious machine, this mock-woman?

OBJECTION THE EIGHTH.

But you who come so late (it will be said) what new discoveries do you bring us? Can you imagine you will, with one dash of the pen, cancel the impression of so many excellent works as have appeared before you? Do you believe a woman can have more ability than so many men of letters, who have labored all their lifetime in perfecting the art, and who so strongly recommend the use of instruments, as the most expeditious method of extricating one self, in all the cases they specify, and where there is a necessity for recourse to extremities? Can you think, that these personages have all spent their time in vain?

ANSWER.

Almost all the sciences and arts attain to perfection, in process of time, through the experience and assiduous attention of those who cultivate them. We owe the most of our rare and precious inventions to the ages of barbarism, in which as yet reigned that brutality and ignorance which the irruption of the northern swarms had diffused over all Europe. This invention and perfection of arts cannot be attributed to merely human industry; but, with more probability, to a particular over-ruling providence, which commonly concealing itself under what seems to us the weakest, and under occurrences which appear to us the effect of chance, have guided men to wonderful discoveries. Do not we owe to a fair Circassian the art of inoculating children? And surely the art of midwifery, perhaps more than any other, stands the fairest chance of being improved by women.

For my part, I dare maintain it, that the surgeons, in form of men-midwives, have been the death of more children, with their *speculum matricis*, their *crotchets*, their *extractors* or *forceps*, their *tire-têtes*, &c. than they have preserved. If in killing the children, they have saved the lives of some mothers, they have hurt and damaged, not to say murdered, a number of others. Their faults ought to set us upon searching out for a better way of going to work; a more easy, a more safe one. This fatal operation by instruments might even be pronounced absolutely useless in the profession. There is no inveighing severely enough against so dangerous a doctrine as that which recommends them. Even common humanity requires an endeavour to open the eyes of those, who imagine they cannot do better than blindly to assent, in every point, to authors recommendable, it is true, by a number of good things, but whose authenticity in those points procures them but the more dangerously credit in erroneous ones. Good sense does not dictate our undistinguishingly receiving all that is advanced even by the best authors. As they may have been themselves deceived, they may also deceive us. The sacrifice of our reason is what we owe to nothing but to revelation. Books written by men have no title to it. As their understanding is not above the impositions of others, or errors of their own, they may adopt falsities, through ignorance, through prejudice, for want of examination, or of right reasoning. Their heart may also have been byassed or corrupted by views of interest or of ambition. I may therefore, without over-presumption aver, that with regard to instruments, it is wrong to lay any stress on the authority of others. For, with all the respect due to some illustrious writers in these modern times, who defend the party opposed to ours, it may be assuredly said, that either they have not known the art of midwifery, or that they have formed their judgment of it by nothing but the abuses of the antients, who practiced it without knowing it. Is it not a crying shame, that operators, who in their life-time massacred such numbers of human creatures, should still retain, after death, credit enough to assassinate common sense? Faith is given to unskillful authors, who have deceived their contemporaries, posterity, and perhaps themselves: ignorance admires, enthusiasm protects them. But what a cruel and mean policy must be that of supposing, that the knowledge of truth ought not to have a clearer title to dominion than the illusions of imposture? I hope however, that, when the eyes of the public shall, in this point, come to be opened, and opened they will be, if true physicians will give themselves the trouble to enlighten it, that public will at length see, that an approbation, unpreceded by a due examination, does it as little honor as service.

Lying-in women principally require an early assistance. For unless they are pregnant of a monster with two heads (a case so rare, that in the practice of a thousand surgeons, in their whole life, it may not twice, nor perhaps once fall in their way) there need never be an occasion of recourse to a surgeon: for in this case, of a monster, it must be the affair of a most profoundly skilled operator and not of merely a common man-midwife.

Run over all the authors who have written on this matter, and you will find that the men-midwives, for want of right, and of true knowledge of the profession, have introduced themselves by force and violence, as one may say, sword in hand, with those murderous instruments: read the antients, it will appear, that they cut their way in, with iron and steel, fore-runners of murders. Our moderns to paliate these violences and injustices, agree on one hand, that the common and gentlest methods are to be preferred: but, on the other hand, when you tell them, that the common and gentlest methods are the hands of women, who ought therefore to be preferred to the men, and to be restored to their antient and rightful possession; then you will see the whole pack open in full cry: to arms! to arms! is the word: and what are those arms by which they maintain themselves, but those instruments, those weapons of death! would not one imagine, the art of midwifery was an art-military?

As for we women, we can but in our weakness groan under this tyranny. Our protest, joined to that of reason and experience, avails little. Our wise innovators have a great deal more wit than we have; but it is not a wit of which we would be ambitious: for it serves them no better, than under the pretence of saving to be paid for destroying: at least it is not unfrequently so.

OBJECTION THE NINTH.

Opinion often makes a stronger impression on us than truth. Whatever you may say to the contrary, the imagination will prevail of life, being safer in the hands of a man than of a woman. For, in short, of what importance can a woman be, who, after all, is but a woman? This is so true, that most of our women now a-days will have a man-midwife, some through prejudice, others through good œconomy, because if there are any prescriptions necessary for the patient, the man-midwife, who is also stiled the doctor, will write for them; whereas, if there is a midwife, a physician may moreover be requisite: this is an additional charge.

ANSWER.

A happiness founded on opinion only, is rather too slightly founded, especially in a point where not less than life is at stake. I know there are women so obstinately wedded to their opinion of certain pretended doctors, that they would not look upon it to be a good office done them, though certainly it would be one, to undeceive them. I also know that the title of doctor is so common in this country, that it ought to be very cheap.

Most of the women in labor, (you say) will have men to assist them, as thinking their life more in safety with them, than in the hands of women. May be so. But what does that prove but the deplorable blindness, the weakness of the human understanding, and the silly prejudices in favor of novelty? Is it then the instruments of these men-midwives that give this confidence or this security? As if a king, a queen, or princess dangerously ill, could be defended from death, by doubling their guards.

The women have on this occasion the delicacy not to suffer even their husband to assist at their labor, and this out of decency. This is very well for those who are contented with midwives; but as for those who will be attended by men to lay them, it is very wrong in them not even to insist on their husband to stay by them. For this preference of men to deliver them, comes either from a greater inclination to the men, or from a greater confidence in them than in the women, or, in short, from the pure necessity they imagine themselves under to employ a man. If it is from inclination, or from necessity, it will always be proper for the husband to stay, to contain the man-midwife, as much as possible, within the bounds of modesty. If the man-practitioner is preferred by them, out of the great confidence they have in men: in what man can they place more confidence than in a tender husband: who more than he can interest himself in the man-midwife's acquitting himself duly of his office?

I wonder that this great confidence which is reposed in the male sex should be limited to the man-midwife only. I promise the women, that they may with equal justice imagine a greater handiness about them in men-attendants than in women; they may just as well have men-nurses as men-midwives: the convenience will be as much greater in the one, as the safety will be in the other. Away then with all the women, who croud round to comfort and relieve a woman in labor: away with your mothers, sisters, aunts or female acquaintance: in consequence to the preference due to the male-sex, let the patient's labor be attended by fathers, brothers, uncles, or men-acquaintance.

But let common opinion lower women as much as it will, so much is certainly and experimentally true, that, notwithstanding the prejudice and superiority of the men, the judgments and decisions of the women are often more shrewd, more exact than theirs. Women have a certain delicacy of mind, which, not being spoilt by undigested studies, renders their taste much more quick, and more to be depended on, than that of the half-learned.

The distribution of merit and talents is entirely in the hands of divine providence, that gives what and to whom it pleases, without respect to the quality of persons; forming out of the assemblage of sciences of all sorts, a sort of empire, which, generally speaking, embraces all ages, and all countries, without distinction of age, sex, condition or climate. The rightful claim to solid praise in this empire, is for every one to be contented with his place, without bearing envy to the glory of others. These he ought to look on as his colleagues, destined as well as himself to enrich society, and become its benefactors. As this providence places kings on the throne for nothing but the good of the people, neither does it distribute different talents to men but for the public utility. But, as in states it has been seen, that tirants and usurpers have sometimes got the upper-hand, so, amongst men of talents there may, if I dare so express myself, creep in a sort of tyranny, which, in the present case for example, consists in looking on the women with a jealous eye, especially those who from an eminence of talents might dispute precedence with them. Thence it is that they are, as it were, hurt by their successes, and by their reputation, and that they endeavour to depreciate their merit, in order to establish the sole dominion in themselves. A hateful defect this, and entirely contrary to the good of society.

This is nevertheless the defect of most of our young men-midwives. But when I consider the mercenary interest by which they are guided, I am far from wondering at their inveteracy against those midwives, especially who are distinguished for their merit and science. The objects of this malignity of theirs are principally those, who have a reputation they fear may enable them to be their competitors in practice. From this mean jealousy of profession, they warmly inveigh against its being trusted in our sex. This is a doctrine they spread every where, and the stale burthen of their abuse is ever, "What is a woman? What effectual service can be expected from a woman?" And thus, by dint of this repetition and of clamor, they come at length to accomplish the persuading an over-credulous public. The common people have in all ages been easily seducible, open to imposition, and when once an error has got full possession of them, it is a miracle if it does not maintain itself in it. They love novelty, are readily taken with striking objects, and stop at the surface of things, which they eagerly seize. Singularity especially moves them. Reason alone, and divested of chimeras, appears too naked to them. They must have something that borders upon the marvellous. Is it not from thence that the dreams of the poets found faith among the Heathens, or that the fables of the Coran pass for so many truths among the Mahometans? To the same weakness in favor of every thing that will make one stare, is owing that silly credulity, which so often leads men to the swallowing the grossest absurdities. One would think fictions had peculiar charms for them.

Nothing however can be more pitiful, than the injustice of running down a sex, which has, in this very matter of midwifery, served the whole earth through all ages, till just the present one, that a small part of the world, becomes in imagination, all of a sudden a land of Goshen, or the only enlightened spot, and takes the ignis fatuus of a mercenary presumption for the sun-shine of sound reason. But after this injustice, where will the men stop? What profession will they leave to the women? It will at last be discovered, that the men can spin, raise paste, cut out caps, pickle and preserve better than we do. After all, is it not even ridiculous to see a custom, established for above five thousand years, universally approved by great and little, fall into disgrace, I will not say by the opinion, but by the whim of a handful of people, most of whom too are, most probably, perfectly sensible of the nonsense and absurdity of that whim, but defend it from a spirit that can hardly not be suspected of interestedness, which indeed will make men defend any thing?

And after all, even common decency and common gratitude might engage the men-midwives to speak less slightingly of the women of that profession; since of whom is it, that the most famous of our present master-men-midwives of London have learned their science but of the women? Do not even the principal ones of them make it their boast to have served a kind of apprenticeship under those midwives, who had served theirs in the Hôtel Dieu at Paris?

But surely the reader will not think it here impertinent to observe, that the wise administrators of that famous hospital, would hardly have failed establishing men-midwives in it, if the safety of the subject had had any thing to fear in the hands of women. But women alone it is that preside at all the lyings-

36

in there, be they never so extraordinary or laborious. The men-midwives have never yet been able to extend their footing within that place. Their emissaries can gain no admission, nor are any proficients trained up there but women only. Notwithstanding which, all the women who are there delivered are satisfactorily and skillfully assisted. Vexatious accidents are less frequent there, in proportion to the numbers, than elsewhere, under the eyes and operation of the men-midwives. Mother and child are both more in safety under the hands of those dexterous matrons, than in those of the most renowned men-practitioners.[3]

To those then, who with a contemptuous tone ask what is a woman but a woman? I shall with equal modesty and truth answer, that generally speaking women are inferior to men in most public services. They are scarcely so fit to head armies, to navigate ships, break horses, or the like, manly employs: but there are certainly domestic branches, in which they rather make a better figure than the men. Midwifery seems their appropriate lot: and rather a gift than an acquisition. They hold from nature herself, in this matter, a certain expertness and dexterity, to which not all the more abstruse refinement of art can ever conduct the men. Nor will the operation of iron and steel instruments ever equal the suppleness, safety and effectual ministry of the fingers of an expert midwife, who understands her business.

Let me then be permitted to ask retortingly in my turn, what is, at the best, a man-midwife? Is not he one of a new set of operators unknown to our ancestors? A creature in short hard to be defined? In no original or primitive language is there so much as a word to express one of this profession. The common word for him in English language is a contradiction in terms, a monstrous incongruity; a MAN-*mid*-WIFE. Sensible of the ridiculous sound of this expression, scarcely less so than that of a *woman*-coach-*man*, they have, by way of remedy, borrowed the term of *accoucheur* from that nation whence the fashion was unhappily borrowed, among many other fashions, so many of which are however rather ridiculous, than like this one *big* with danger, added to the ridicule of it. But even that affected French word *accoucheur* is of a very recent date in France. No French authors employ it, who are not themselves of a more modern date than the word itself, which has not above the antiquity

---

[3] The Commentator on Boerhave's Lectures, vol. V. p. 252. or §. 694. says, "*At Paris women are taken into the Hôtel Dieu, fifteen days before their lying-in, at the public expence, so that the business of midwifery can be no where better learn'd.*"

of a century to boast. The name and vocation of a midwife are found in the most primitive languages, being, in fact, coeval with mankind itself.

As to those who, from a principle of œconomy, prefer a man-midwife to a midwife for conducting a lying-in, with respect to the remedies and prescriptions which may be necessary on those occasions. Œconomy is doubtless a laudable consideration, but I am much afraid, that those who on this occasion make it a reason of preference, much mis-calculate things. This man-midwife you prefer is either an eminent or an ordinary one. If he is an eminent one, you are not always sure of having him in the greatest need; for besides their being so rare, they cannot be every where at one time. But admitting that you are fortunate enough to fall into the hands of a man-midwife of the greatest name in the profession, can you imagine that you will have a very cheap bargain of him? These gentlemen expect no small fees, and will not attend without them. You would besides be ashamed of not doing honor to the footing on which they give themselves out. Whereas the same gratitude is not always shewn to a midwife, however skillful in her profession, and whatever trouble she may give herself both before and after the lying-in of her patients; notwithstanding too the assiduous attendance and visits she bestows upon them till they are out of danger; notwithstanding these tender attentions she has for the children, which are so seldom regarded by the men-midwives; there are who imagine they cannot give a midwife of this sort too little, and that for no other reason on earth, but because she is not a man.

If on the contrary, and what the most frequently happens, you fall into the hands of one of the common men-midwives, either of that multitude of disciples of Dr. Smellie, trained up at the feet of his artificial doll, or in short of those self-constituted men-midwives made out of broken barbers, tailors, or even pork-butchers (I know myself one of this last trade, who, after passing half his life in stuffing sausages, is turned an intrepid physician and man-midwife) must not, I say, practitioners of this stamp be admirably fitted, as well for the manual operation, as for the prescriptions? If then it is from thrift they are employed, by way of sparing fees to a real physician, I own, I think this is pushing savingness too far; as I should be almost as much afraid of the prescriptions of these mock-doctors as their operation. I should have more confidence in the advice of a discreet matron, or of a skillful midwife, who, by habit and a long experience of seeing ladies in their lyings-in attended by the best physicians, is in the most common cases of the labor-pains, more able to advise the sick person to innocent remedies, where there is no complication in the disorder, than those half-bred or ignorant pretenders: but if there is a complication, then there must absolutely be a good physician called in, the expence of which should not be regretted, since life is at stake.

Now in such cases, a midwife, though never so skilful, will neither be ashamed nor backward to require such aid: whereas a man-midwife, the more ignorant he is, will be but the more careful of concealing that ignorance, and from the most false prejudice that both the faculties of physic and surgery are implicit ingraftments on the profession of midwifery in a man, will rather let mother and child perish, than call in that assistance, of which he will be ashamed to confess his standing in any need. He will then rashly do the best he can for his patient: but what will that best most probably be? Torture and death; and that with perfect impunity. I say most probably, for not even the most credulous, or the most zealous for the appropriation of this profession to the male-sex, can hardly carry the blindness of credulity and obstinacy the length of assenting in earnest, that in the common run of men-practitioners you are to find at once the man-midwife, the physician, and the surgeon. Whereas women, fully sufficient for all cases but the very extraordinary ones indeed, are ever ready to call for proper help, on the first alarm of danger, of which too their apprehension is much more quick and just than that of the men.

OBJECTION THE TENTH.

The ignorance of the women is the cause of the little confidence there is reposed in them.

ANSWER.

If this objection was fairly stated, it should be said, that the ignorance of the women in the art of destroying mother and child, occasions their not being trusted so much as they deserve with the office of saving both. In that art indeed of perpetrating double murder with perfect impunity, under the sanction of the public credulity, imposed upon by a vain parade of learning, I readily confess the men superior to the women. I do more than confess it, I will prove it; and how? Even from their own writings and confession, not extorted from them by the spirit of candor, but from an interested desire of decrying or supplanting one another, in order to self-recommendation.

In fact, whoever will, with a competent degree of knowledge of the subject, and of due impartiality, peruse the practical treatises of midwifery, written by the most celebrated practitioners, some of whom have so vainly pretended to the triple union of the characters of man-midwife, surgeon and physician in one person, and it will be found, that all their boasted superiority of erudition, has only led them into the greater errors of practice, and the most barbarous violences to nature.

But perhaps I exaggerate. Let the reader judge for himself, and pronounce as his own reason shall dictate to him. Let him if he can read without shuddering, the following quotation from one of the most celebrated *men-midwives* of the age, Levret, p. 199. "Mauriceau had invented a new *tire tête*, which was to be introduced into that part (the uterus). Peu or Pugh, like *many* others, made use of different hooks (*crochets*) and La Motte opening the head with scissors, scooped out the brain, &c. We read, with horror, in *all* these authors, that they have extracted children, who, tho' much *maimed* or *mutilated*, have yet *lived* several hours."

Upon this many reflections will naturally occur. These children thus destroyed, owed most probably their death neither to nature, nor to the difficulties of the passage through which the launch is made into our world, but to the labor being prematurely forced, and the delivery effectuated by those torturous instruments, which at once kill the child, and not seldom irreparably wound the mother in the tender contexture of these parts. A midwife, with less learning and more patience than those gentlemen, and well acquainted with the power and custom of Nature to operate in some subjects, sometimes more slowly, and in all ever more safely and gently than art, would have left to nature, not without her tenderest assistance of that nature, the expulsion of the child. A proper predisposal of the passage, and direction of the posture, with an unremitting attention to employ the fingers, so as not to lapse the critical moment of operation, often never to be recovered with safety to mother and child, would have, I repeat it, and appeal to common sense for the probability thereof, saved the lives of those innocents, which thus fell the victims of those *learned* experiments, with instruments, which, by the way, be it remarked, none are so forward to use, as those who are the loudest in exclaiming against the employ of them. And reason good, if they exclaim against them, it is evidently in order to cover their practice with them, against which the minds of their patients must so naturally be revolted. But that exclaiming does not evidently hinder their being used, when, the truth is, that if due care was previously taken with the patients, those execrable substitutes to the fingers need never be used at all.

But if these instrumentarians were called to account for their so justly presumable massacres, what would be their defence? Most certainly not the truth. One would not own, that in order to attend a richer patient, or perhaps to return to his bottle, he had recourse to his fatal instruments, to make the quicker riddance or *effectual* dispatch; another would not confess, that he employed them purely because his fund of *patience* was exhausted, some would not care to allow, that they used them purely on the scheme of trying experiments; and none of them would, you may be sure, plead guilty of ignorance of better and more salutary methods. No! their wilful error, or that major skill, they would be sure to conceal under the cloud of hard words and scientific jargon, in which they would dress up their respective cases, and insult the ignorance of those silly good women, who *know* no *better* than to deliver those of their own sex with the help of their fingers and hands, and who are so undextrous, as to have no notion of putting them to such unnecessary tortures and risks, as are inseparable from the use of those iron and steel instruments. Instruments which rarely fail of destroying the child, or at least cruelly wounding it, and never but injure the mother, not only in those exquisitely tender-textured parts, where they are so blindly and ungovernably introduced; but in the often irrecoverable dilatations of the external orifice, the vagina, and especially the *fourchette* or *frænum labiorum*, all which, in general, they considerably damage: and always originally without necessity. For if through carelessness, if through an impatience, so much more natural to men than to women, in a case and position of this nature; if through ignorance of the critical minute of extraction, the occasion of operating with the fingers has *not* been *lapsed*, any recourse to instruments is perfectly unnecessary, and they will hardly ever succeed where the subject is inaccessible to the fingers, without having the worst of consequences to dread from them both to mother and child. Nothing then can be worse for a man-midwife, than to be tempted to any negligence, to any precipitation, to any ostentation, in short, of expedition or of superiority of skill to that of the women, by his having those instruments at hands, the doing without which is at once so much better and safer, even by the confession of those who use them nevertheless.

How greatly then is the ignorance of the midwives preferable to *such* an use, as the male-practitioners commonly make of that deep learning of theirs, which only misleads them, at the expence of humanity! How over-compensated is that want of theoretical knowledge, so unjustly reproached to women, since they possess a sufficiency even of that knowledge; how over-compensated, I say, is that supposed want, by that instinctive keenness of apprehension, and ready dexterity of theirs in the manual operation, which in them is a pure gift of nature, and to which not the utmost efforts of art or experience can ever make the men arrive, for reasons which will be made clearly appear in the two following considerations.

First, It will hardly be denied, that the art of midwifery requires a regular training or education for it. The season of that education can only be that of youth. And surely in that season precisely, the very nature of the study excludes those of the male-sex, at the same time, that there is nothing in it indecent or improper for the females destined to that profession. This proposition will be more clearly illustrated, by an appeal to the reader's own sense and reason upon what passes, and must necessarily pass in those hospitals for the reception of lying-in women, where those of the male-sex are allowed to attend for the sake of learning the profession.

This Charity is indeed founded upon specious motives, but the conduct of it would make humanity shudder, even where no violence is expressly intended to humanity; and without the least forced or uncharitable conclusion, may serve to demonstrate the impropriety of attempting to throw the practical part of midwifery into the hands of male-practitioners, the implicit consequence of which must be the exclusion of the midwives, without any direct and formal exclusion of them, but purely from the discouragement that will hinder any good and able ones being formed in future. And that no thorough-good men-midwives, except perhaps two or three extraordinary men in a whole nation, can ever be formed, the procedure at the lying-in hospitals, open to men-pupils, such as it must of all necessity be from the nature of the thing itself, without any the least reproach herein meant to the worthy managers, will convince all who will make an unprejudiced use of their judgment.

We will then suppose a lying-in hospital, in which, for the sake of training up *men* to the profession of mid*wives*, there are young pupils of the male-sex admitted to attend and learn the practical and manual part of the business. To obtain this end, we will not say that women of virtue and character are subjected to the inspection and palpation of a set of youths, who perhaps pay largely for their privilege of attendance; but we will grant, that the objects of this charity are entirely women, who, though they may have unfortunately forfeited their right to virtue, cannot however have lost their claim to the protection of that humanity, which, besides the great and most political attention due to population, pays especially a tender regard to the innocent burthen, though of a guilty mother. Yet among these wretched victims, there may be not a few who, if they were not even to deserve more compassion than blame, for particular circumstances of their ruin, in which the villainy of men has often a much greater share than female frailty itself, cannot surely deserve that all traces of modesty, or natural remains of regard for it, should be utterly eradicated by that hard necessity of theirs to accept of a charity, by which they must be abandoned up to the researches of a set of young men, to whose approaches their age and sex must alone give an air of petulance and wantonness not to be explained away, to the satisfaction of the poor passive sufferer, by the goodness of the intention. Every one must be sensible of the dreadful effects such a treatment must have on the mind of a poor creature in that condition, when the imagination is known to be the most weak, and susceptible of the most dangerous impressions. At that critical time, amidst all the terrors and apprehensions inseparable from her situation, she is moreover exposed to the greatest indignity that can be well imagined, that of serving for a pillar of manage to break young men into the exercise of that most unmanly profession. Nay, that very circumstance of the use she is put to, which she is in fact to consider as a kind of valuable consideration by her paid for the relief afforded her, and which in that light can scarce be called a charity; that very circumstance, I say, of her submission, at all calls, and upon all pretences of the pupils, being accounted for to her by the good intention of it, will yet hardly pass on a wretched, frightened, harassed woman, who, whatever may be said to procure her tame acquiescence, can scarcely, if she has a spark of female modesty lest in her, be reconciled to the grossness of such usage, whether she considers herself as the butt of wantonness, or the victim of experiments, or perhaps of both the one and the other. It is well if she is defended by her ignorance from any idea of those dreadful instruments, of the having practices tried upon her with which, her circumstances might but too reasonably render her apprehensive, since a needless resort to them may be too often presumed in the course of practice, where the men are even paid for their assistance. These the men-midwives may possibly indeed conceal from the sight of their patients, but I defy him to conceal them from their wounded imagination, if they are not wholly ignorant or can think at all.

Yet in pure justice to all parties it should be observed, that, besides many other points to be learned only by ocular inspection and manual palpation, of which no theory by book or precepts can convey satisfactory or adequate notions, that great and essential point in our profession, a skill in what we call the *Touching*, is not to be acquired without a frequent habit of recourse to the sexual parts whence the indications are taken. And in this nothing but personal experience can perfect the practitioner. But this admitted, only proves the more clearly the utter impropriety of men addicting themselves to this occupation. For, once more, most certainly the season of acquiring the nicety of hat faculty of *Touching*, besides other requisites in the art, is for obvious reasons that of youth. Now let any one figure to himself boys or young men, running at every hour, and exercising a kind of cruel assault on those bodies of the unfortunate females, upon which they are to learn their practice. But will they learn it by this means? It is much to be doubted. It may perhaps be granted, that men of a certain age, men past the slippery season of youth, may claim the benefit of exemption from impressions of sensuality, by objects to which custom has familiarized them. But, in good faith, can this be hoped or expected in the ungovernable fervor of youth? Can such a stoic insensibility be imagined in a boy or young man, as that he can direct such his researches by pawing and grabbling to the end of instruction only? Must not those researches, humanly speaking, be made in such a disorder of the senses, as to exclude the cool spirit of learning and improvement? May he not lose himself, and yet not find what was the occasion of losing himself? In short, granted, though it is surely hard to grant, that the wretched women, admitted to this so falsely called Charity, may not deserve much tender consideration; but in what can the poor young pupils have deserved so ill of their parents or guardians, as to be thus exposed to temptations so shockingly indecent? What father, what mother, what considerate relation can paint to himself a child, or charge of his, at an age so incapable of resisting the power of sensual objects, as is that of youth, employed in exploring them too in vain? It is surely easier to guess the natural consequences, than to defend either the subjecting youths to them, or the hoping any good from the subjecting them. In short, even Dr. Smellie's doll is a more laudable method of instruction.

But besides this reason taken from the moral impossibility of laying a timely foundation of practical knowledge in the male-sex, for preferring women under the false charge of ignorance, to the so unconsequentially boasted learning of the men, there remains a yet stronger argument against the male-practitioners: an argument furnished by nature herself, and of the which, every impartial reader's own feelings will in course render himself the judge.

Nature has to all animals, from the man down to the lowest insect, to all vegetables, from the cedar to the hyssop, to all created beings, in short gives what is respectively necessary for them. Nor can it without the grossest absurdity be imagined, that this tender universal parent, or call her by a yet more sacred name, the divine providence, would have failed women in a point of so great importance to them, as that of the ability to assist one another, in lying-in, at the same time, that she has given them so strong and so reasonable a sympathy for those of their sex in that condition? Can it be thought that nature, so vigilant, so attentive, to the production of fresh generations, through all beings, should have been deficient or indifferent as to women, her favourite work, the friend, the ornament of human kind? And so she must have been, if she had left her in the necessity of recourse to others than those of her own sex, in whom there exists so sensibly a superior aptitude for tending, nursing, comforting and relieving the sick, that even the men themselves, in their exigences of infirmities, can hardly do without them. But to say the truth, and as I have before remarked, nature has been even liberal in her accomplishments of those of the female sex for this office. Not content with giving them a heart strong imprinted with a particular simpathy for their own sex, on this occasion, a simpathy, which for its tenderness, has some

45

resemblance or affinity to the instinctive love or *storge* that parents have for their children; she has also bestowed on them a particular talent, both for the manual function in the delivery of women, and for all the concomitant requisites of their aid during the time of their lying-in: a talent in short, which may even be felt, without the necessity of definition or proof, to be superior to any possible attainment of the men in that art, though they should have sacrificed hecatombs of pregnant rabbits, or have brooded over thousands of coveys of eggs in their search of excellence in it. To say nothing of a certain softness, flexibility, and dexterity of hand, palpably denied to the men, there is, both in the management of the manual operation, and in the attendance due on those occasions, a quality in which the women, generally speaking, excel the men, and that is, patience, a quality more essential, more indispensable than can well be imagined. For on patience it is, that the salvation of both mother and child often depend; whether that patience is considered in the so needful point of predisposing the passages, or of waiting, without however over-waiting, the critical efforts of nature in the expulsion of her burden. Now nothing is more certain, than that nature, who to woman has in general given all that vivacity and quickness of spirit, which seems incompatible with the phlegmatic quality of patience, has, as if she had purposely meant an exception favourable to her darling end, the propagation of beings, especially the human one, bestowed on the female sex, such a remarkable assiduity and diligence in aid of womens labors, as are rarely to be seen in men, and when seen, appear rather forced than naturally constitutional to them. Women, in those cases, have more bowels for women: they feel for those of their own sex so much, that that feeling operates in them like an irresistible instinct, both in favor of the pregnant mother and of the child. Thence it is, that a woman-practitioner will employ, without stint, or remission, all that is necessary to predispose the passages, for the least pain, and the greater safety; she will patiently, even to sixteen, to eighteen hours, where an extraordinary case requires so extraordinary a length of time, keep her hands fixedly employed in reducing and preserving the uterus in a due position, so as that she may not lapse the critical favorable moment of extraction, or of assisting the expulsive effort of nature: and what man is there, can it be imagined, would have endurance enough to remain so long in a posture, the very image of which, in one of his sex, is so nauseating and so revolting, to say nothing of the want of that pliability and dexterity of management of the fingers, and those occasions, so necessary, and so uncommon in the men, especially in that very age; when their practice should be supposed the greatest.

It is then in those cases where nature is slow, as she sometimes is, in her operation, and often so, for the greater good of the patient, so conformed perhaps, that a quicker expulsion would only destroy her, that the midwife, not only uses all patience consistent with safety of life to the mother especially, but inculcates patience to her suffering charge. Whereas *the men*, from their natural impatience, or from whatever other motives their precipitation may arise, having those infernal iron and steel instruments at hand, are but too often tempted to make use of them, not only without necessity, but against all the indications of nature, pleading for a just indulgence to her of her own time in her own work. In vain then do too many of them declaim as loudly as can be wished, or as the thing deserves, against all recourse to instruments, but in extremities which, they pretend, justify them. In the first place, those extremities are often the fault of deficient and unskillful practice. The precious moments of the assistance due to nature have been lapsed, or there has been some failure of preliminary treatment; or what is worse yet, extremities are rashly taken for granted when they are not existing.

Here, in the history of one single woman, I give the history probably of thousands.

A healthy woman, about twenty five years of age, and remarkably robust, was in labor of her second child. Her first had come in that natural smooth way, as had given the same man-midwife, who was now to lay her again, not the least trouble, as often happens. In this second labor, however, the head of the child stuck in the passage; and was so far advanced, that the Doctor told her, whether in jest or earnest I cannot say, that he could discern the color of its hair. Her pain, though extremely great, had not however hindered her observing the Doctor rummaging for his instruments; her frightful apprehension, of which, she had all the reason to imagine, did not a little contribute to retard her throws. She taxed him with his intension to use them, and he did not deny it. Upon this she used the most moving fervorous entreaties for a respite of execution; but all in vain; he told her, with a resolute tone, that he knew surely better what was for her good than she did, that he

47

had even already waited longer than he could justify; and that her life was absolutely desperate if the child was not instantly extracted, of the which being dead, he was sure from many incontestable symptoms. Her thorough confidence in a man, whom she had often heard declaim vehemently against the use of instruments unless in extremities, and which she understood in the most literal sense, without considering, or perhaps knowing that, on too many occasions, nothing is so different as words and actions; her thorough confidence in him, I say, joined to a natural love of life, and to her present feelings of exquisite pain, determined her to an acquiescence. The fatal instrument was struck into the brain-pan of the child, who at the instant gave the lie to the first part of the Doctor's asseveration as to its death, by such a strong kick inwards as had almost killed her, and convinced her not only of its being alive but lively. This did not, you may be sure, add to her belief of the second part of his averment, that waiting any longer for the operation of nature, would infallibly have been her death. It might be so: yet surely there are strong reasons for concluding, that a little more patience might have saved a fine boy, and yet not have destroyed, or even hazarded the destroying the mother, whose life is certainly the preferable object. But how cruel to state the dreadful alternative where it does not exist! And how easy, in the presumption of that alternative, to extort the dreadful consent from a weak women, yet more weakened by her condition, and naturally determined by her present feelings, to embrace the appearance of an immediate relief, presented to her in the form of salvation of life! However, scenes similar or a-kin to this, may, without breach of charity, be presumed too frequent, especially under those super-ficial men-midwives, whom he facility of forming, in the manner they are generally formed, renders so suspicious as to their ability, and who for so many reasons, both of nature and interest, are but too liable to the murderous want of that patience, for which the women are but the more remarkable in this case, for their not being perhaps so capable of it in any other. But here their duty is even their nature; as if in so capital a point, she would trust it to nothing but herself.

If it should be here to this objected that the women may, through that very spirit of patience, wait too long, or overstay the time of saving the patient's life, for want of calling in proper assistance; I have already implicitly obviated this objection, by remarking before, that a true thorough midwife, from her quickness of apprehension, and knowledge of the danger, will ever be readier to call in the assistance and advice of a physician, than the common men-midwives, who are ever in proportion to their ignorance the more rash, the more fearless, and consequently averse to calling in that help, of which they will be ashamed to confess their want, and thus cruelly, though with impunity, lose the opportunity to others endeavouring at least to repair those damages, of which themselves are oftenest the authors. Now a midwife has no such shame; she pretends to no extraordinary skill in physic or surgery; she knows her art, and will not presume to transgress its bounds; she would think herself accountable if she did: and even that very tenderness and sensibility, upon which nature has founded her patience, will make her cautious how she pushes that patience too far. She may easily see, feel and discern those cases in which nature calls the physician in aid to the midwife; nature, who seems to have placed such boundaries between those professions, as nothing but interest, presumption, or ignorance of nature, could ever render their union in one person supposable: tho' the quality of physician may not indeed exclude that of the surgeon, but rather implies, at least, the theory of surgery. For I presume anatomy is the great basis of true rational physic, though it can very little assist practical midwifery, which depends so much upon purely manual operation, and needs only sufficient general idea of the structure of the sexual parts in woman, the conceptacle, and passages of the delivery.

This is so true, that any impartial observer of the male and female practitioners in midwifery, will easily distinguish the characteristic difference of the sexes, in their respective manner of operation.

In the men, with all their boasted erudition, you cannot but discern a certain clumsy untowardly stiffness, an unaffectionate perfunctory air, un ungainly management, that plainly prove it to be an acquisition of art, or rather rickety production of interest begot upon art.

In women, with all their supposed ignorance, you may observe a certain shrewd vivacity, a grace of ease, a handiness of performance, and especially a kind of unction of the heart, that all evidently demonstrate this talent in them to be a genuine gift of nature, which more than compensates what she is supposed to have refused them, in depth of study, though even of that they are not so unsusceptible, as some men detractingly think; and in midwifery, most certainly they attain all that they need of learning to perfect them, with a facility the greater for nature, having collaterally endowed them with an organization of head, heart and hand, obviously adapting them to this her most capital mystery. This will be denied by none who have any regard for truth, and who do them justice, as to the keenness of their apprehension, as to that sympathizing sensibility which supplies them with the needful fund of patience, and tender attention; and as to that peculiar suppleness of the fingers, as well as slight of hand, in a function which rather exacts a kind of knack or dexterity, than mere strength, of which they have also a competency. Nor can it be quite without weight, that the midwives, besides their personal experience, being sometimes themselves the mothers of children, have a kind of intuitive guide within themselves, the original organ of conception, itself pregnant, in more cases than that, with a strong instinctive influence on the mind and actions of the sex; an influence not the less certainly existing, for its being undefinable and unaccountable, even to the greatest anatomists.[4]

The men, it will be said, have many or all of these qualifications, except indeed the last. Granted that they have: but how very few are of the men that possess the most essential ones to a degree comparable to that of the women: or rather not so imperfectly, as that all their boasted skill in literary theory and anatomy, cannot supplement or atone for the deficiency? Nor theory, nor all the books that ever were written on that subject from the divine Hippocrates,

---

[4] It is evidently this universal influence of the *Uterus* over the whole animal system, in the female sex, that Plato has in view in that his description of it, which Mr. Smellie (introd. p. 15) calls odd and romantic, from his not making due allowance for the figurative stile of that florid author. Thus the diffusion of the energy of the *uterus*, Plato calls its "*wandering up and down thro' the body.*" A power of activity which, towards conquering the otherwise natural coldness of the female constitution, nature would hardly give to the uterus merely to excite in woman a desire, sanctified under due restrictions, by her favorite end, that of propagation, if she had not, at the same time, endowed that uterus with an instinct, beneficial by its influence in the preservation of the issue of that desire. And the real truth is, that there is something that would be prodigious, if any thing natural could be properly termed prodigious, in that supremely tender sensibility with which women in general are so strongly impressed towards one another in the case of lying-in. What are not their bowels on that occasion? It may not be here quite foreign to remark, in support of the characteristic importance of the uterus or the womb, that in the antient Saxon language the word *Man* or *Mon* equally signified one of the male or female sex, as *Homo* in Latin. But for distinction-sake the male was called *Weapon-man*, (not however for any offensive weapon or instrument in midwifery;) and the female *Womb-man*, or man with an uterus: from whence by contraction he word woman.

50

who understood so much of physic, and so little of midwifery, down to Dr. Smellie, who is so great a man in both, will ever amount to so much as the practical experience of a regular bred midwife.

As to that superior skill of the men in anatomy which is sounded so high, against the women, I shall not imitate the men in their want of candor towards the female-sex in their availing themselves of false arguments. I will not then take the benefit of the slight opinion which Celsus and Galen had of the depths of anatomy; they who contented themselves with a gross superficial notion of the principal viscera. I will not even desire to countenance that contempt by the example of that great philosopher Mr. Lock, the intimate friend, and even the counsellor of the British Esculapius Sydenham, who paid a great deference to his physical knowledge; and yet this very Mr. Lock wrote an ingenious treatise (though not published by him) upon the insignificance of the refinements of anatomy in the practice of physic. Neither will I here insist on the absurdities into which even the greatest anatomists have fallen; as for example, *Pecquet*, the famous discoverer of the thoracic duct in the human body, who nevertheless adopted so extravagant a notion, as that digestion of food ought not to be promoted by exercise, but by drinking spirituous liquors, a practice to which himself fell a victim, dying suddenly at the anatomical theatre. It is only for those who have a false cause to defend to shut their eyes against those truths which seem against them. Those on the contrary who defend purely the truth, know that one truth cannot hurt or exclude another truth, and that all truths may very well coexist. It may be true that anatomy, though it does not give the nature of the elementary composition of parts intrinsic and too minute for the human sense, since a new incision only presents a new surface, much conduces however to ground the student in mechanical principles of great assistance to him in practice, of which they are doubtless the most solid foundation: yet that truth is not incompatible with another quite as much a truth, that midwifery can have no occasion but for a general notion of the configuration of those parts upon which it is exercised. A midwife, for example, may be a very safe and a very good one, without knowing whether the uterus is a hollow muscle, or purely a tissue of membranes, arteries and veins: but if that ascertainment is necessary, she must wait for it till the anatomists have settled among them that point, which, like many other capital points of anatomy, is not however yet done. In short, once more, a woman in labor required a midwife to lay her, not an anatomist to dissect her, or read lectures over the corpse, he will be most likely to make of her, if he depends more on the refinements of anatomy, than on the dexterity of hand, and the suggestions of practical experience and common sense.

If then, there are who can examine things fairly and with a sincere desire of determining according to the preponderance of reason, they cannot but on their own sense of nature, on their own feelings, in short, discern that no ignorance, of which the women are undistinguishingly taxed, can be an argument for the men's supplanting them in the practice of midwifery, on the strength of that superiority of their learning, so rarely not perfectly superfluous, and often dangerous, if not even destructive both to mother and child. Consult nature, and her but too much despised oracle common sense; consult even the writings of the men-midwives themselves, and the resulting decision will be, that great reason there is to believe, that the operation of the men-practitioners and instrumentarians puts more women and infants to cruel and torturous deaths, in the few countries where they are received, than the ignorance of the midwives in all those countries put together where the men-practitioners are not yet admitted, and where, for the good of mankind, it is to be hoped they never will.

I have here said few countries have hitherto countenanced men-midwives. That I presume is too notorious to require proof: for even those Saracen or Arabian physicians, Avicen, Rhazes, &c. who, by the by, are little more than servile translators or copists of the Grecian ones, wrote only theoretically in quality of physicians; for it does not appear that they ever practised midwifery themselves, nor ever got the practice of it by men introduced into their countries. Among the Orientals there is no such being known as a man midwife: that refinement of real barbarism, under the specious pretext of humanity, is happily unknown to them. But if it should be said, that the jealousy so constitutional to the inhabitants of the warmer climes, has a share in the exclusion of men-practitioners; the women have, at least in that point, a weakness to thank for its production to them of so great a good, as the greater safety of their persons and children, in that capital emergency of their lying-in. For, after all, the art of midwifery is, in the hands of men, like certain plants, which, by dint of a forcing culture, exhibit more of flourish, or a broader expansion; but besides ever retaining a certain exotic appearance, they never come up to the virtue of those spontaneously growing in the full vigor of a soil of nature's own choice for them. Art may often indeed improve nature, but can never a supplement to her, where she is essentially wanting. Deep learning may, in very extraordinary cases perhaps, repair the errors, or assist the deficiencies of the manual function, but the deepest learning will never bestow the manual function, nor indeed can in the same person exist, but at the expence of the manual function, which must have been in some measure neglected for it. And yet the greatest practical skill that any man can with the utmost labor and experience acquire, will hardly ever equal the excellence in it of the women, Great Nature's chosen instruments for this work: an excellence by them attained with scarce any learning at all, or at least of that abstruse theoretical sort, on which the men make their superiority principally depend.

But that I may not herein be taxed of maintaining any thing that has only the air of paradox, or of begging the question, I shall implicitly, in the course of my answer to the following objection, endeavor to remove any remaining doubt on this head.

OBJECTION THE ELEVENTH.

In like manner, as there are particular parts of the human body which have their appropriate undertakers or protectors under their proper distinctive names, as oculists, dentists, and corn-cutters, who by making respectively one part their particular care and study, arrive at a greater perfection, at least in the practical operations on it, than regular physicians or surgeons, whose object is the whole fabric; Why, by parity of reasoning, should not the men-practitioners in midwifery be preferable to the midwives, since a man has to his manual function super-added a theory superior to that of the women, who, it is confessed, stand sometime in need of calling in the physician to their assistance? As a man then will have laid in a stock of medical knowledge, peculiarly adapted to the exigencies and disorders incident to women during their pregnancy and lying-in, he must consequently excel the midwife, or the physician singly considered; he who with so much greater convenience will have united in one person both their faculties, besides that of the surgeon.

53

That certain parts of the human body enjoy the protection of practitioners, who respectively devote themselves to their service, I confess. Such appropriations may also be beneficial, at least, to the practitioners. I can even conceive, that a professed dentist may clean, scale, and draw teeth, or an oculist couch a cataract, better than either a physician or surgeon. These may in their respective practice be excelled by those partial artists. But I much doubt, even as to these, whether their trusting too much to that partial excellence, does not sometimes do more mischief than good, for want of duly consulting the relation of such parts to the universal fabric, of which physicians and surgeons must be so much better judges. Galen does not appear in contradiction to common sense, where he observes, that to rectify a disorder of the eye, the head must be rectified, which cannot well be done without rectifying the whole body. In confirmation of which, I once myself knew a gentleman, whom a professed oculist, at Paris, assured of the loss of his eyes being infallible; and who upon his despondingly consulting a regular physician, was by him as positively assured, that those very condemned eyes might be saved by a proper regimen. The gentleman happily believed him, and his eye-sight was not only saved, but perfectly restored.

Another instance of the like nature occurs to me, which seems applicable to the dentist, and which I quote here from a translation of the learned and ingenious Dr. Huxham's observations on the constitution of the air.

"Many years ago I knew a gentleman of a hale, robust habit of body, who, from being too much addicted to the drinking of brandy, fell into a violent jaundice, from which however he would have recovered well enough, would he have conformed himself to the advice of his *physicians*: but he on the contrary, because his *gums* were very apt to bleed, and his *teeth* stunk from the *scorbutic taint*, put himself into the hands of an ignorant *pretender to physic for the cure of these inconveniencies*. This fellow immediately set about *scaling his teeth*, and *rubbing his gums* with *his famous teeth-powder*, till at last, by perpetually fretting and irritating the loose texture, he brought on such a hemorrhage, that baffled all the stiptics that could be invented by the most expert surgeons, and continuing to spout forth in small streams from the little arteries of the gums, which were now every where divided: in the space of *sixteen hours* the poor man *died* through mere loss of blood."

These instances are however only adduced to justify that doubt which I expressed of these partial artists being *always* to be beneficially consulted in those local affections, to which their talent is supposed exclusively appropriated.

Corn-cutter is indeed a homely plain English term, but if the teeth give from the Latin the appellation of dentist, as the eye that of oculist, what name, taking it from the *part* in question, will remain for that language, to give the men-practitioners of midwifery, in substitution to that hermaphrodite appellation, that absurd contradictory one in terms, of *man*-mid*wife*, or to that new-fangled word *accoucheur*, which is so rank and barefaced a gallicism? But let what name soever be given them, it can hardly be too burlesque an one, considering the gross revolting impropriety of men, addicting themselves to a profession naturally so little made for them.

Paint to yourself one of these sage deep-learned *Cotts*, dressed for proceeding to officiate[5], and presenting himself with his pocket-nightgown, or loose washing wrapper, a waistcoat without sleeves, and those of his shirt pinned up to the breasts of his waistcoat; add to this, fingers[6], if which not the nicest paring the nails will ever cure the stiffness and clumsiness; and you will hardly deny its being somewhat puzzling, the giving a name to such an heteroclite figure? Or rather can a too ludicrous one be assigned *it*?

Those however who will consider this grave Doctor in his margery field-uniform, this ridiculous piece of mummery, in a light of seriousness, such as

---

[5] Smellie. Treatise of midwifery, p. 339. *where it appears, that the above dress is reserved for a man-midwife's masquerade-habit in private practice, before ladies, not to frighten them; whereas to the poor women in hospitals his looking like a butcher, is it seems necessary, with bases and an apron; the* steel *of course.* But if it is not too presumptuous for me to offer so *learned* a gentleman as the Dr. a hint of improvement for his man-practitioner's toilette, upon these occasions, I would advise, for the younger ones, a round-ear cap, with pink and silver bridles, which would greatly soften any thing too masculine in their appearance on a function which is so thoroughly a female one. As to the older ones, a double-clout pinned under their chin could not but give them the air of very venerable old women.

[6] *If a man happens by great chance to have long taper fingers, it is a circumstance so uncommon, that it is proverbially said of him, "He has rare* midwife's *fingers."* Nor was it quite unhumorously observed of one of the founders of the sect of instrumentarians in England, remarkable for a raw-boned coarse, clumsy hand, that no forceps he could *invent* of iron or steel, being more likely to hurt than his fingers, he had, at least, that excuse for recommending instruments.

the matter perhaps more justly deserves, especially combining with all the rest, the idea of his crotchets, forceps, and the rest of his bag of instruments, may think he less resembles a priestess of Lucina, than the sacrificer, in a surplice, with his slaughtering-knife, to one of those heathen deities whose horrid worship required human victims, which the poor lying-in women but too nearly resemble.

But whether or not, in imitation of the dentist, or oculist, he receives his title from the particular part he has taken under his protection, so much is certain, that the same arguments, which militate for those partial artists claiming their respective departments of the human body, will not avail the man-midwife. An oculist, a dentist, a corn-cutter, have no operations to perform but those of which disorders equally incident to both sexes are the object. There is nothing in their practice repugnant to the nature of the male-sex, nor to that reasonable decency, which only requires that no sacrifices of it should be made in vain, or at least not made to no better a purpose than to increase at once the danger and the pain of both mother and child, in whose favor it is sacrificed, as it may be clearly proved to be oftenest the case. But of the chirurgical part of the man-midwife's pretention, I reserve to treat after considering him in the capacity of a physician; in which a man may indeed be wanted, but in that of surgeon never, or at least so very rarely, as not to atone for the dangers which attend the men forming themselves into a set under the name of men-midwives.

Where there is no complication of any collateral disorder with the gestation and parturition of women, it is even a jest for men to pretend the necessity of any study or practice to which women may not arrive, and even much excel them.

But where there exists the case of a singular constitution, or of symptoms declarative of other help being necessary than just the common one, that quickness of discernment, that peculiar shrewdness of the women, in distinguishing what is relative to their art from what is foreign from it, gives them the alarm in time, and if they have a just sense of their duty, or but common sense, they must know that such disorders cannot be *partial*, cannot therefore be considered as they are by the man-midwife, as subordinate to his particular province, relative as they are to the whole fabric or system. All *partial* practice then is here absolutely out of the question, and now what help can, consistently with good sense, be expected from a man-midwife, who, under a natural impossibility of ever acquiring the female dexterity in the manual operation, cannot however, be supposed to attain even that imperfect degree of skill, without sacrificing to the endeavours at it the time and pains in study and practice, which are requisite to form the able physician?

But, in fact, the men, that is to say, those of that sex who have the best understood all the refinements of anatomy, all the variety of female distempers, never that I can learn, attempted to invade the practical province of midwifery. The immortal *Harvey, Sydenham,* the great *Boerhave, Haller,* and numbers of others who have written so usefully upon all the objects of midwifery, have never pretended or dropped a hint of the expedience of substituting men-midwives to the female ones. They contented themselves with lamenting the ignorance of some midwives, from which has been drawn a very just inference of the necessity of their being better instructed; but even those great men never chose the character of practitioners themselves, nor probably would have thought it any detraction from their merit to have it said, they might make a bad figure in the function of delivering a woman.

Whoever then will consider but how the common run of men-midwives actually are and must be formed, and assuredly the number of exceptions to the general insufficiency cannot oppose the interference, must allow that, where a woman has distempers collateral to her pregnancy, with which they must also become dangerously complicated, she must expose herself to the utmost hazard, in any confidence she may place in a man-midwife.

The truth is, that most of the dangerous lyings-in are so far from being likely to be relieved by a man-midwife, that it is often to the having relied upon his medical judgment, and especially to his manual skill they are owing. But of the first only it is we are now here speaking.

The women captivated by that assiduity of the men-midwives, of which they only fail when they are not paid or likely to be paid, in some form or other, up to the value they set upon themselves, lightly take for granted, that, as men, they are also capable physicians. It is enough, in short, for these practitioners not to be women; for the women to think they can prescribe for them in all disorders. A mistake this, often big with the utmost danger to them.

The men-midwives, in general, have never, at the most, carried their studies beyond the disorders commonly incident to pregnant women: the knowledge of all the other possibly collateral ones, is what even the least modest of them will hardly claim, unless to the profoundly ignorant, and is in fact scarce less than impossible to one who has applied himself essentially to the manual function. In such cases the ignorance of a midwife can hardly be greater than that of the men-practitioners, and must be less dangerous from her less of pretention. Her consciousness of her own want of sufficient light, will engage her readily to state the exigency to some able and experienced physician, whom she must allow, in such cases, to be her superior judge: whereas the other, the man-midwife, acknowledges no greater authority than that which he is pleased to invest himself. He stands, in virtue of a distinct business, and a business for which he never was made, of a sudden the self-constituted sovereign dictator and inspector-general of all female disorders whatsoever, where the woman is with child, that is to say, where the case is only thereby rendered much the more nice and difficult, and, not rarely, does he continue under the same pretext, to extend his practice to where there is no pregnancy at all in the case. And yet ask him for his titles, they are all implicitly dependent on or subordinate to that same mid-wifery, for which he is so naturally unqualified, even if a due study and exercise of it would permit those avocations, that would contribute to accomplish him in the so necessary general knowledge of physic. But indeed why need he acquire it, since it is so commonly taken for granted, or that he is believed upon his own word, especially if he is backed with a diploma, for form's sake, that may have cost him little or nothing of medical study, or indeed of any thing but the amount of the fees for it?

Yet how serious, how important is it for women, if they tender their own lives, and that of the previous burthen of which they are the depositaries, to make that distinction between the physician and the midwife, which they seem so little to make! How little do they consider, what nevertheless is strictly true, that a man can never at the best be but an indifferent practitioner of midwifery, though he may be an excellent one in physic; but that as bad a midwife as he can be, he must be yet, if possible, a worse physician, if he attempts to throw both professions into one, and exercise them jointly! They are incompatible, from the justly presumable impossibility of one man doing justice to the practice of the one, unless at the expence of the study of the other: by which other, to obviate cavils, I repeat it, I mean the general practice of physic, which comprehends the speculative part of midwifery, as well as all other branches understood to be the province of the physician. This distinction then I make, because, as to the diseases purely incident to pregnant women, experimental practice will rather assist the medical study of them: and it is in that part only the men-midwives can make any figure at all, and that not a superior one to midwives who are regularly bred, and who have, in their favor, their excellence in the manual function besides.

Once more, in complicated cases, the most dreadful mistakes are to be dreaded from those common-men-midwives, who so groundlessly erect themselves into physicians on those occasions. A purge, a venesection, or any other prescription injudiciously ordered, may be the occasion proximate or remote of death to both mother and child; yet a woman, at least, *ought* not to expect better from one of these practitioners who, for the most part, has neither study nor experience in general physic; nor more than a smattering of anatomy, joined to the index-learning of dispensatories. Such a man-midwife can never have thoroughly made himself master of the course of the fluids, nor of the order of their circulation. Their relation to the solids, and the efficacy of medicines upon both, can hardly be sufficiently known to a man, who must have been too much employed in trying to form a hand never to be formed, and in attendances on the practice of his midwifery, to acquire those collateral requisites for the effectual multiplication of his professions.

Yet this man void of knowledge, experience, observation, and, in consequence, of physical ability, shall boldly decide on the expedience of an internal remedy, of which he does not know the power or operation; of a venesection, of which he can but guess at the consequence; and of a narcotic, of which he is unaware of the danger. In all which, observe, he may possibly sometimes be tolerably right, in cases where there is *no* complication; that is to say, in cases when a midwife, duly bred, is as sufficient as the best man-practitioner. But then she is moreover not only quicker of apprehension, as to danger, where the case appears complicated, but readier to call in proper help where she discerns it to be above her reach, and consequently above that of the man-midwife, who must be equally or rather more at a loss, because his boasted theory will serve only to puzzle him, or what is worse yet, since a shew must be made of doing something, *will* most probably determine him improperly, if not fatally, to random prescriptions, in points out of his sphere of knowledge, or rote of practice.

Many a man who to-day undertakes prescribing for a fever, for a fit, a convulsion in a lying-in woman, only because he appears in the character of a man-midwife, would have been ashamed the day before he had taken up that business to give himself out for a physician. He would have been afraid of ordering any thing for her if she was not his patient, as to lying-in, and would not, even after assuming the profession of midwifery, perhaps order any thing for the same woman, out of the time in which his office is supposed necessary. This plainly proves, that many of those gentlemen are weak enough to imagine, that the man-midwife implies the physician, though the greatest physicians that ever were never dreamt of such an absurdity, as that the physician implied the midwife, whose master and instructor he rather is, in points highly useful indeed at times to her profession, but in which that profession does not consist.

I do not however charge *all* the men-midwives with so much modesty, as to confine their striking out of midwifery into physic, to the women lying-in, or to the time of their lying-in, since there have not been wanting some who, with equal ignorance, but superior effrontery, have intrepidly hoisted, the standard of a general knowledge of physic, and having originally insinuated themselves into families in the character of men-midwives, have easily maintained their ground in them afterwards on the foot of physicians. A circumstance not much to be wondered at, considering the endearment of such an office as that of a man-midwife, and the ascendant it must serve to give them over the heads of families, even in points where a midwife can have no shadow of pretention, for interfering. In the mean time, let any one of sense or common humanity consider but the consequences of this dangerous admission of the sufficiency of a man-midwife in those complicated cases, which require the consultation of a regular physician; to say nothing, for the present, of the other objections already mentioned, or which I shall hereafter more at large discuss, and the result must be, to allow that the medical pretentions, or indeed any pretentions, of these men-practitioners, cannot be too much discouraged, nor confidence more mis-placed than in them. For once that they may hit the mark by chance, they will often take the part of the distemper instead of that of the patient; they will do what they have only a gross guess of being the right, not what they know to be so: and physic, at best, but a conjectural science, must in them want even the common grounds of conjecture.

Instead then of the dangerous self-sufficiency of these complex smatterers, you have in a plain midwife, supposing her regularly bred, and duly qualified for her profession (for I am no more an advocate for ignorance in the women than in the men) one, who, being called in time, will duly consider, and observe the constitution of the person that wants her assistance. If nothing appears extraordinary, or out of the common-rules in her patient's constitution and conformation, she needs only lay down for her the previous course of management, and as the hour of delivery approaches predispose her properly: a point in which the men must be grossly deficient, for want of that skill of prognostic inherent to the women, from their particular delicacy and shrewdness in the *faculty of touching*; upon which more depends than can be well imagined. Wherever a case occurs to a midwife, so complicated as to be above her reach, her interest, her reputation, her duty, all conspire to prescribe to her a timely application to a regular physician. She communicates her doubts or difficulties to him, who, at the same time that he receives a just information from her of the state of things, combines it with his own knowledge of the human constitution. He does not confound, as the man-midwife does, ideas so different as those of the manual operation, and the medicinal prescription. The object of the physician, being the same as that of the midwife, the prevention or alleviation of pain to the mother, and the greatest safety to the mother and child, but preferentially that of the mother; there is this advantage to both mother and child, that all harshness of practice, all the violenter remedies will be as much corrected as can be done, consistent with the safety of mother and child, by the midwife's tenderness, by which the physician will at the same time be above the being misled into omissions of any thing absolutely requisite. In short, on such occasions, they serve to temper on another. A truly great physician will not disdain the lights furnished him by her practical experience, and she knows the bounds of her mechanical duty and profession too well, to interfere with his superior intellectual province, in those points submitted to it. A pragmatical man-midwife, on the strength of his miserable half-learning, would think it a derogation from his character, to call in a physician in supplement to his deficiency, of which he is always ashamed, though indeed he has sometimes the excuse of himself not knowing it. Then when a fatal accident has happened, under his hands, against which, with more knowledge he might have guarded, or which with less of presumption or dependence on himself he might have prevented, by procuring previous or collateral advice; he thinks himself abundantly acquitted by laying the blame on *occult causes*. Even the great man-midwife, *Mauriceau* himself, has made use of that trite exploded apology[7]: where he expressly says, "that a sudden unexpected death of his patient was one of those FATALITIES, that not all the human prudence can prevent."

But that I may not here incur the least charge of unfairness, as if I meant by this quotation any thing so absurd or unjust, as that in the labors of pregnant women, as well as in other diseases unconnected with them, there may not sometimes happen accidents impossible to be foreseen, as well under the care of the best physician, called in by the very best midwife, as under the most ignorant assuming man-midwife, I shall here introduce another quotation from the same *Levret*, that will especially shew the ladies, and all parties concerned, to what an imaginary safety, so much, and even the very point sought for, is sacrificed as is sacrificed, in preferring the men-practitioners to the midwives.

[8]"M. de la Motte says, that for the fifth time he laid the wife of a glover of Valogne, the 16th of March, 1704; that the woman was but an hour in her labor-pains, and that he delivered her with all the facility imaginable; that he left her upon the couch till he had given her some broth, after which he recommended her to the care of the nurse, and went *where his business called him*. He adds, that he had time but just to bleed two persons in the neighbourhood, before he was fetched away in haste to see the patient he had just laid, whom he found *dead* upon the bed. The cause of this *death* was instantly manifest to him from the stream of *blood*, which ran about the floor, and even penetrated to the apartment beneath, after soaking through the bed itself, in which there remained clots of blood of an extraordinary size.

"This author adds, in the reflexions at the end of this observation, that this delivery had been both more easy and more expeditious than any this woman had precedently had: and he notes, that these *melancholic accidents* are not

---

[7] *A la verité* Maureveau *raporte cette mort inopineê à une* CAUSE OCCULTE, *puisqu'il dit expressement que* "ce fut un de ces fortes de malheurs de la destinée que toute la prudence humaine ne peut pas eviter." *C'est aussi l'opinion de* la Motte. LEVRET, p. 272.

[8] Levret, p. 269.

without example, since such ladies as the princess of —— and madam la Presidente de —— with *numbers* of *others*, have, on the like occasion, undergone the same *fate*, as her he here treats of. These are, according to him, *proofs* that all human science and dexterity *often* cannot prevent the *like misfortunes*, since these *great ladies* had been lain by the most *celebrated men-midwives*."

Now I might here, without much probability of being contradicted, aver, that where such accidents, said to happen so *frequently* and inevitably, should happen under the hands of midwives, there would be but one voice among the men-practitioners and their credulous adherents, to impute them to the ignorance and malpractice of the women. The plea of *occult causes* would be hooted at in them, tho' receivable, it seems, from the men.

Not however to imitate what I condemn in them, a gross want of candor to the women, of whom, by the by, the very best of the men-practitioners have learnt all the laudable part of practice, I shall allow that among those frequent examples, of sudden deaths upon delivery, some few might perhaps be of those unaccountable surprizes with which nature mocks human ignorance; but then it must be allowed too, that not all of them admit of that favorable solution. The truth is that nature, to those who have studied her course, and watched her motions with a due spirit of practical observation, hardly ever but gives warning enough to prepare proper obviative methods. It is not here the place to enter into the discussion of those deaths by sudden hemorrhage upon delivery, of which I shall hereafter attempt to give a more satisfactory account, as well as of the measures of prevention, than Levret. My end in the preceding quotation is to show;

First, that by the confession of the men-midwives themselves, the most fatal accidents *frequently* and *inevitably* happen under them in spite of all their *science* and *dexterity*!

Secondly, to offer to the reader a reflexion for himself to judge of the validity of it, to wit, that, not only in the cases of the hemorrhage, but in many others, where there is a complication of disorders with the state of pregnancy and parturition, much of the safety of mother and child must depend on that general medical knowledge, to which the men-midwives have so little grounds of pretention. Nor indeed, for the symptoms of necessity for resorting to medical help, have they the same shrewd prognostic or acute sense as the

63

experienced women, who much sooner perceive the danger before it is too late, and are neither with-held by a false shame, nor by a criminal or senseless presumption, from calling in proper assistance. Such at least has been and still is their practice in all ages, and in all countries, where the matters of pregnancy and lyings-in are committed to them. The great object of the man-midwife is to impose so false a notion on his patient, as that his partial knowledge is sufficient to every thing. The consequence of which is, that if he is not too officious, too pragmatical, by way of ostentation of his art, in common cases, that is to say, where there is no complication of disorders, every thing may pass off tolerable well, till the crisis of labor-pains. And in that crisis I defy him, with all his learning, to equal the female skill and cleverness, not only for lessening the sufferings of the patient, but for facilitating the happy issue of her burden.

But where there is a complicated case, dependent on the physician's art, then the trusting to those men-dabblers in midwifery is a folly that may be fatal to both mother and child, or, at the best, the delivery will have been rendered more painful, more laborious, more big with danger, for those precautions having been neglected, which can be so little supposed to occur to the common run of men-midwives in cases foreign from their rote of practice. Yet it is precisely in those disorders collaterally contingent to pregnancy, and no disorder does that state exclude, that the greatest skill and knowledge of physic are required. Then it is, that not only the preservation of the mother claims regard, and certainly the preferable one, but even that of the child is no indifferent point. And to save both, the state of the mother's constitution must be carefully considered. Thus the combination of the disease with the pregnancy, the due regard to the mother as well as that to the child, form a triple object that takes in a compass of comprehension to which no midwife will pretend, nor can be imagined to exist in the mere man-practitioner of midwifery. Such a nicety of observation does not seem to be the province of a manual operator, and indeed useless to him in that character. And as he will be more likely to trust to conjectures, which no sufficient grounds of study will have justified his presuming to trust, he must oftener take the part of the disease than of the patient. It is well if sometimes, disconcerted at the excess of a danger of which he does not understand the origin or nature, he does not, in default of the head, employ the hand, and engage the mother in a premature or forced delivery of the child, to the imminent hazard of the lives of both. Now comes the chirurgical operation in play; and we shall now see, that the ingraftment of the surgeon upon the midwife, deserves equally at least reprobation with that of the physician.

But before I enter on this disquisition, I am to observe, that this objection to the surgeon's commencing midwife, does not in the least attack the merit of that respectable body of men, the surgeons. No one can honor their profession more than I do: I even readily grant, that their skill in anatomy is of service to midwifery itself, into which it throws a great light. It would be easy for me to name, if requisite, several surgeons, who are not only an honor to their country, from their excellence in an art so beneficial to mankind, but an ornament to society, from their extensive humanity and charity. These, I am so far from thinking, will hold themselves honored by the men-midwives attempting to make a common-cause with them, that I rather depend on their bearing witness on the part of the women in this cause, which is indeed the cause of Nature, of that Nature which they study so practically, consequently so usefully, and with which they are so conversant. I am persuaded they can even furnish me with arguments, from their superior store of knowledge, in supplement to my deficiencies. The surgeons must look on these professors of midwifery as a kind of amphibious beings, hard to define, whose claim exhibits rather the deformity of a preternatural excrescence, or wen growing out of the chirurgical art, than the becomingness of a natural member of it. Most of the first founders of this new sect of instrumentarians in this country were, or I am greatly misinformed, neglected physicians, or surgeons without practice, who in supplement to their respective deficiencies, greedily snatched at the occasion at that time of a prevailing whim in France, of employing men-midwives, with just such a rage of fashion, as some of the ladies there prefer valet-de-chambres to waiting maids. This novelty then appeared to practitioners despairing of business enough in their own way, an excellent scheme for eking out their scanty cloth with this bit of a border, of which by degrees they have made to themselves a whole cloak. In short novelty joined, to the much exaggerated objections to perhaps a few insufficient midwives, brought in and established a remedy yet worse than the disease. Their success encouraged others; and now behold swarms of pupils pullulating, and forming on the models before-mentioned. Thus two or three maggots have produced thousands. Iron and steel are not tender: and yet it was by the pretended necessity of resorting to instruments made of these metals, that these out-casts of either profession effectuated their introduction into a business so little made for them. Then it was, that not with the least squinting view to filthy lucre, but purely out of stark love and kindness of the women, that these redressers of wrongs, armed with their crotchets, and other weapons of death, took the field on the hardy adventure of rescuing the fair sex out of the dreadful hands of the ignorant midwives. But as to the validity of that plea of theirs, of the necessity of employing instruments; I reserve to treat of it at large in its place in my second part.

Here I shall only request the reader to remember, what has been said of the indecent, superficial, and even cruel method of training up pupils in this upstart profession. But if I was to add here my having been credibly informed, that there are novices who watch the distresses of poor pregnant women, even in private lodgings, where, under a notion of learning the business, they make those poor wretches, hired for their purpose, undergo the most inhuman vexation, in a condition so fit to inspire compassion, and where those scenes must be rather a school of brutality than of art: if I was to urge, what from the great probability of the thing I firmly believe, that more than one unhappy creature has fallen a victim to the rudiments of these novices; that especially not long ago, one of them in a hurry and confusion of presumption and ignorance, instead of the after-birth from a woman, tore away, by mistake, her womb itself, which occasioned, of all necessity, the poor creature's dying in unutterable agonies of torture: if I was yet to go farther and assert, that even not one of the least eminent men-midwives pulled off the arms of a child in his attempt to extract it, and very gravely laid them upon the table; what would be replied to me? It would be said I had invented these horrors, or forged such raw-head and bloody-bones stories, purely in favour of my own cause. And to this objection, while I produce no proof, and for my producing no proof other reasons may be obviously assigned, besides that of those cafes being non-existent, some of which I am very certain are true, and firmly believe all the rest; to this objection then I say, I make no reply. The reader, who will have considered this matter, may easily decide within himself the degree of probability in such allegations. But what objection will stand good against authorities of reasonings and facts, produced from the writings of the *men-midwives* themselves? Will they be suspected of partiality or aggravation of things against themselves?

I shall here select one of perhaps the most excusable examples from the circumstances accompanying it, or it would probably not have been produced by the author a man-midwife, to shew, by the confession of the men-midwives themselves, the insufficiency of their discernment, whether a child is dead or not.

"Edge-tools and crotchets naturally inspire horror, and though they *ought* not to be employed unless on a dead child, it is well known the mother is not always *safe* from the effect of them. Besides there are *no signs* of the death of a child, though he should have stuck in the passage for several days ... *certain enough* to authorize a recourse to a method which infallibly *kills* it, if it is not dead before. This is so true, that whoever will turn over the authors antient and modern, on this subject, there is not *one* of them that gives us *satisfaction* on this point. On the contrary, they *all* seem *agreed* on the *insufficiency* of these signs, and there are even *few* of them who do not bring examples to support this uncertainty.

"Here follows one taken from the observations of Saviard, p. 367. This author says, that a chirurgical operator, whose name he *prudently* suppresses, being sent for in aid of a midwife[9], to extract a child that had stuck six days in the passage, and which he *thought* dead, from several of the signs most essential to conviction, it happened however, that having opened with his *bistory* the teguments and membranes which occupy the as yet unossified space, at the commissure of the parietal bones with the fontanelle, it happened (said he) that an opening this place with his bistory, introducing his crotchet at this

---

[9] This will doubtless be laid hold of as one proof, that midwives have, in cases where they are puzzled, been forced to have recourse to men-practitioners: but I have no where said, there were not some midwives unequal to their business. The sequel will shew, that this most probably was one of them, and the case was not much mended by the assistant she called in. A little more patience, though I confess there is some room to think it in this so long lingering case excusably exhausted, would have prevented the murder of the child: but as the concomitant circumstances are not specified, I cannot pretend to determine that point. All I shall say is, that there is not hardly one case in a thousand, in which nature does not know her own time best, and does not take it kindly to be hurried. It has been known, that sometimes the quickest deliveries have been the most fatal, and the most liable to sudden death, by consequent hemorrhages.

opening, and having fixed it in one of the parietals, he drew out the child, who began to cry *piercingly*, all hurt as he was by so *large* a *wound*, that there came out of it more than an egg full of its *brains*, which made a *cruel* sight in the eyes of the by-standers, and a very mortifying one for the operator.

"It were to be wished that this was the *only* example: but I will not relate any *more*; it is easy to think one cannot be too *circumspect* in the matter of such relations. Levret, p. 77."

Now I, who have not the same reason for *circumspection* in this case, as Monsieur Levret, with strict regard both to matter of fact and to candor, *agree* with *him*, in averring, that this is not the *only* example perhaps, by thousands, of the rash resort to the expedient of *opening* the head, and extracting the child with the crotchet; an expedient which, as Dr. Smellie observes, (p. 248.) "*produced a* GENERAL CLAMOR *among the women, who observed, that when recourse was had to the assistance of a man-midwife, either the mother or child, or both were lost.*" Now of not filling up the cry of those women, I must own I should be most ashamed. Especially when the good Dr. by way of curing our fears and *weak* apprehensions, and of shewing the nonsensicalness of them, first very gravely tells you the insufficiency of *all* hitherto invented instruments, and only modestly concludes, that the forceps of his own ingenious contrivance, is indeed the best, but still imperfect. His homage to truth would however not have been so imperfect, as it is if he had said that instruments may be totally left out of good practice, and that no "*artificial hands*", as he calls them, can, in any case, constitute a worthy supplement to the *natural* ones; no not even to his own, supposing iron and steel to be ever so little less tender than his fingers.

[10]But why do these gentry then so much insist on the absolute necessity there is of *sometimes* having recourse to instruments?—Why? The motive for that insistence is so transparent, that not to see through it would indeed be blindness. It is the capital, and perhaps the only plea that has the least shadow

---

[10] Dr. *Smellie* has himself (p. 403.) ranked among the causes of sudden death to women by violent floodings after delivery the following one; "if in separating the placenta the accoucheur has scratched or tore the inner surface or membrane of the *womb*." But if unpared nails, or the rough hands of a man, may cause such a dreadful accident, what may not be dreaded from iron and steel instruments, blindly thrust into parts of a scarce less tender texture than the apple of the eye? But of that more hereafter.

of plausibility for the men to intrude themselves into the women's business of midwifery. The women do not pretend to the art of handling those instruments, and would be very sorry to pretend to it. Nor do those midwives, who are sufficiently skilled in their art, ever need the supplemental aid of them: whatever is done with them is as well, and infinitely more safely done without them: so that the only grounds of introducing men into that female practice is essentially false. The making then the surgeons art a pandar to a sordid interest, by the incorporation of midwifery with it, is, in fact, engrafting on a noble stock, a scion of another one, both which would bear very well separate, but, thus joined, can produce nothing but a vile poisonous fruit.

If there could be such a thing as laughing in a matter of such general importance to human kind as the fixing of this point, there could hardly be any refraining from it, with regard to the conduct of the men-midwives, especially in Paris. There the novices of them, sensible of the natural defect there must be in men-practitioners, apply for improvement to the regular midwives. There is particularly, among others, one Madam Clavier, who when I knew her, lived in the Rue de St. André, that gave lessons, at so much a-head, to the men-students of midwifery. Yet these same men have no sooner got a smattering of all that is valuable in the profession, for beyond a practical smattering at most nature refuses them further progress; they, I say, have no sooner acquired a little useful insight from these laudably communicative midwives, but they are the first to swell the cry against them of, "oh these *ignorant midwives!*"—or *"what can be expected from a woman?"* And what is more yet, among women it is, that they can make this equally ungrateful and false clamor prevail. And women, in a point of the utmost importance to themselves, prove that the men have, in fact, not quite a wrong idea of their weakness, since they are weak enough to countenance a notion, that so unjustly dishonors them in every sense. But that is not enough. What one should imagine, women especially would consider, is that this notion received with its consequential exclusion of those of their own sex, tends to have their own pains aggravated, and the safety not only themselves but of their so naturally dear children, yet more endangered.

For the truth of this increase of pain and danger from the practice of the instrumentarians, it is not to any representations from me only, who may be supposed too interested a party, but to reason, and even to reason's best mistress, Nature herself, that I appeal. I appeal even to the very writings of the most celebrated men-midwives themselves, to which I would refer all who are sincere enough with themselves to be resolved to embrace truth when discovered to them. It is then even in the writings of those men-practitioners, that a lover of truth might find enough to satisfy himself, that all the mighty pretences of the men-midwives to superiority of skill and practice to the women are false and absurd. Look into *Deventer, Peu, La Motte, Mauriceau, Levret, Smellie,* &c. and you will find that, except their accounts of the *innocent* manual function, in which midwives must so much excel them; except *their* pernicious practical part, on which they so tediously insist, by way of recommending each some particular instrument that is to *usher* him into employment, and increase his profit, in which noble view he takes care to decry the instruments of all others, or at least prefer his own; except the scientific jargon of hard Latin and Greek words, so fit to throw dust in the eyes of the ignorant, and give their work an air of deep learning; except what they have pillaged from regular physicians and surgeons, who have treated upon these matters: except in short all the quacking verboseness of the various histories of their exploits and deliverances of distressed women, and you will find the merit of their whole works shrink to little or nothing, under the appraisement of common sense and true practical knowledge. The most that you will find in them, is, hard or lingering labors, oftenest precipitated fatally to the mother, or at least to the child; they hardly, you may be sure, carrying their candor so far, as always to mention when it has proved so to *both*; of which however the tenor of their practice with instruments gives you but too much room to presume the probability. In short those cases, of which their works are chiefly patched up, are little better than so many quack-advertisements; and their best exploits therein recounted not a whit preferable; nor indeed so practically just, as what would appear in the common daily practice of a regular well-bred midwife, that should keep a register of her deliveries. There might not indeed appear so much anatomy in her descriptions, but, I am very sure, there would be couched in them much more solid instruction. Not that I therefore have not the highest deference to the true physicians, the true surgeons. But as far as I can presume to judge, it is not in the works of the men-midwives, that the best lights in midwifery are to be looked for. They are themselves for every thing that is worth reading in their writings indebted, both to the physicians and surgeons, whose arts they have despised enough to think, they may be well enough learnt collaterally and subordinately to the mechanical operation of midwifery, as well as obliged to the midwives, to whom they *ought* at least to go to school, tho' sure to rail at their *ignorance* the minute after being taught by them. In short, the most valuable lights thrown into this subject are undoubtedly furnished by those great men Boerhave, Haller, Heister, the great Harvey, and other the like excellent physicians and surgeons, not one of whom however, I presume, in the way of making a trade of it, ever delivered a woman in his life.

Nay! was any accident requiring a chirurgical operation to befall a pregnant woman, I should think the application would be more safely made to a thorough regular-bred surgeon, than to one of the common run of these men-midwives; and the exceptions are so few, they are hardly worth making. The reason too for such a preference is obvious and natural. A regular surgeon probably would not only be more consummately skillful and expert in his general notions, both theoretical and practical, so far as surgery was in the question, but would not, from any thing only *partial* in his profession, have the same temptation of bringing into play a horrid apparatus of murderous instruments, to show the importance and utility of that anatomical midwifery of theirs, all the art of which consists in the violences it offers to Nature. What would be to be done, the true surgeon could hardly do worse than the pragmatical man-midwife, and most probably would perform it much more artist-like, except perhaps in the sole point of striking a crotchet into the brain-pan of a live-child, or needlessly tearing open, with iron and steel, parts so tender and so delicate, as hardly to bear the touch of even the softest hand, guarded with all precaution. He would not, in short, be so forward to use means destructively dangerous to both mother and child, and at the best often to ruin a woman for being a mother for ever after.

Upon the whole then, if any one will dare give his own understanding fair play, against the powers of prejudice and interested imposition, it cannot but, on a fair examination satisfy him, that that strange anomalous complex creature of the three arts, physic, surgery and midwifery, is most likely to excel in neither. IT may by great chance be an indifferent physician; it must be in this respect a dangerous surgeon, but IT can never be any thing but a

71

despicable midwife; or if that favorite name of *accoucher*, IT is so fond of assuming, should not be popular enough from its gallicism, let IT change it for the Latin one of *Pudendist*: a word of not one jot a more pedantic coinage than *Dentist*, or *Oculist*, but of which moreover the propriety of the sound may somewhat atone for the pitiful play of words it contains, and which can yet scarcely be more pitiful than the object of its application.

Objection the Twelfth.

It is not probable, that the men-practitioners would have come into the vogue in which we see them, if numbers of instances were not to be produced in their favor, of their having terminated happily many labors, in which they have been preferably employed, and to the exclusion of the midwives.

Answer.

This only proves, what none in their senses will deny, that the greater part of the cases of labor are so mild, that not even that faultiness of the men-practitioners, which is palpably owing to an incurable imperfection of Nature, not, in short, all that is bungling or deficient in their preliminary disposition and manual operation, can absolutely frustrate the kindness of that Nature, of which these intruders are not ashamed of assuming the honor. But that inference of the men in favor of themselves is as ridiculous as it is false. In those cases of labor, which are much the less frequent, and require no extraordinary assistance, the utmost of the real merit of these bunglers is only of the negative kind: that is to say, they have not destroyed the mother nor the child; and indeed, every thing considered, great is the praise to them thereof. It is not always, even in naturally easy labors, that the women who employ men to lay them have not a harder bargain of them.

But even in these propitious labors, the mischief done to a lying-in woman, by employing of a man to the exclusion of a midwife, is not a small one, if pain is an evil, and the lessening that evil a desirable good. For certainly there can hardly be a case of lying-in supposed, in which some *labor-pains* are not felt. The bringing forth children in pain, stands hitherto the irreversible decree of nature, from which few women can promise themselves a total exemption.

But these pains, if they cannot be entirely spared, to the lying-in woman, will always admit of actual or preventive alleviation. That alleviation can be no inconsiderable object to women, who are by their nature so tender and so impatient of pain. Even then in the prospect and presence of the very gentlest labors, there are two natural points to be respectively attended to. The one is the predisposition of every thing, according to art, so as to render the expected labor-pains as moderate as possible. The second is in the manual function, at the actual crisis of the delivery. Now, in both these points, for reasons above-deduced of the superior aptitude in women derived to them from Nature herself, a woman may reasonably depend not only on a more sympathizing cherishment, but a more efficacious assistance from those of her own sex. There are a thousand little tender attentions suggested by nature, and improved by experience, that a midwife can employ both preventively and actually to the mitigation of her charge's pain; attentions which, if even they ever entered into a man-midwife's head, could not be accepted but with repugnance, I will not say only by a modest woman, but by any woman at all. And the truth is, that there can be few men in the world, but what, the more tender lovers they are of the women, but must be only the more disgusted, the more impatient of the midwife's preparatory part of her office, which is however the most important one, both as to the prevention of pain, and to the safety of the delivery.

But even where those preparatory offices have been omitted, or at best perfunctorily performed by a man-midwife, and where the actual function in the crisis of labor has been deficient, or at best indifferent, the labor may still have proceeded, and the patient delivered with only more pain, than she would probably have suffered under a good midwife's hands. What follows then? Why this; that the patient in the transport of joy at her delivery from pains which are hardly ever but great, even though much less than her fear had magnified them to her; instead of gratitude to that Nature, which can constitute to her only a vague object of the mind, her weak imagination gives to the assistant man-midwife, a more palpable being, as he is of flesh and blood, the merit of a deliverance, in which he had most probably no other share, than its being his fault that it was not yet less painful than she has found it. But this is not at all. What sounds towards a paradox, and yet is strictly true, is, that the more pain the patient has endured, through the man-midwife's fault, the greater will her gratitude be to him. The reason is as obvious as it is natural. Herself not knowing, nor having perhaps any idea of what ought to have been done for her more perfect relief, she will have no conception that the man has omitted any thing: she will give him credit for what he has *appeared* to do for her; and measure her sense of acknowledgement by the pain from which she will suppose he has helped to rid her; and in her joy at her delivery would think it even an ingratitude to listen to suggestion from others, or even from herself, that should tend to diminish, explain away, or may be reduce to less than nothing, the benefit she so vainly imagines was his work.

Yet nothing is more true, nor indeed more likely to be true, than that besides the natural pains of labor not having been obviated by a due prevent method of assuagement; besides their having been unskilfully attended to in the article of the delivery, through the natural unhandiness of the men-midwives, it does not unrarely happen, that their defective practice, not only occasions to the women much greater pains, but even much greater danger than would probably have been the case, I will not say if a midwife, but even if Nature had barely been left to herself, that is to say, if nature had been neither injured by a clumsy aukward attempt to help her, nor injudiciously interrupted, nor prematurely forced or cruelly hurried. The patient is however delivered, and delivered so that, if she was better informed, or less blinded with joy, instead if thanking the operator, to whom she attributes her deliverance, she would have to impute to him all the increase of pain she had unnecessarily suffered, all the increase of danger of which this man so thanked was himself the author. Then it is, that even in a subject so serious, a judicious by-stander might give himself the comedy of observing the airs of consequence, which an operator assumes for a woman under his case *not* losing the life, of which but for him she would most probably *not* have been in the least danger. Thus a man, whose all of merit well weighed, is no more than not having been able to consummate the destruction of mother and child, in spite of the kindness of nature, shall for that negative merit be allowed the positive one of having performed wonders of art. Then it is that the mother naturally in a rapture of joy at her deliverance, in which she never remembers but with a gratitude, of which she only mistakes the object, by paying to the operator, what in fact was due to nature; then it is, I say, that the mother, father or parties concerned, for want of making due allowances in a point they are so excusable for not

74

understanding, cordially join the self-applause of the man-midwife. Nor does it unfrequently happen, that one of these instrumentarians, after an operation, for which he deserves the severest censure, and of which, whatever necessity he had to plead was originally owing to his own unskillfulness or omission, shall strut about the room, and flourishing his butcher's *steel*, sing an *Io Peean* to himself, *"for that his victorious art had saved nature as it were by enchantment"*[11]. Then it is, that in full chorus the deluded parties, in the innocence of their heads and hearts, hold up their hands to heaven, and piously exclaim, *"what a narrow escape the patient had, thanks to the learned Dr. and what a mercy it was she had not been trusted to such an ignorant creature as a midwife must be."*

This folly has even sometimes gone so far, that when a woman has, through a man-midwife's mis-practice, suffered perhaps a wrong, so deep as to be disqualified for ever after for being a mother, or had a fine child, literally speaking, murdered (*secundum artem* indeed) he has, what with scientific jargon, through the cloud of which it was impossible for persons unversed in the matter to discern the truth, what with an air of importance, and what with especially her own weak prepossession in favor of the superiority of men to women-practitioners, known how to impose on her the most atrocious injury for so great a service as that of saving life is for ever held. The deceived patient then thinks she cannot thank him too much, nor reward him sufficiently for what he could be scarce punished enough, if proportionably to the mischief he had done; and to which his mis-representations have perhaps even made herself innocently an accomplice;

This indeed is easily to be accounted for. A pregnant woman must especially, in the moment of her labor-pains, think herself too much in the power of the operator, to whom she has trusted herself, to dispute his judgment. She may even, and that is probably oftenest the case, have too good an opinion of it, to dispute it. Her labor is severe, and, as before observed, severe, or at least the more so, very likely from some fault of his. Her deliverance lingers; Nature, from some vice of conformation, or defect of art in her assistant, appears faint, remiss, insufficient, in short, in her expulsive efforts; in the mean time, the pains of the patient grow more and more intense

---

[11] Levret's words, p. 279.

and intolerable: the man-midwife, either perplexed or impatient, or not knowing what better to do, has recourse to those fatal instruments, with which the odds are so great, that he will gall, bruise, or irreparably wound the child, or the mother[12]. In some cases indeed, he may take the dreadful advantage of the mother's agonies of pain, to use those instruments, and do her a mischief she may not just then feel, from the pain of the operation being absorbed in the greater one; to use them, I say, unobserved by her[13].

But where the exigency appears yet greater, where, in short, the operator imagines, as he too often imagines such an extremity where it does not exist, as that either the mother or the child must perish, it is his maxim, and certainly a very just one, to consider the mother's safety, as the preferable object. Of this preference then he makes a merit, so much the more acceptable to the mother for her own self-preservation being so palpably concerned, and so much the less disputable for her not knowing but he may be in the right, as to the reality of the fatal dilemma. In such a doubt, if nature takes the part of the child's life, which is at stake in the decision, she also much more strongly and reasonably takes the part of the mother's own existence in the mother's own breast. She cannot then deny the premisses, of which she is no judge, when the inference is not only in favor of her life, but even a very just one upon the admission of those premisses. The temptation also of a quick riddance from a violent state of pain, is too great a temptation for a weak woman, overpowered with her actual feelings in that rack of nature, to resist: she acquiesces then, or perhaps her husband, her friends, equally ignorant with herself of the truth of things, and duly sympathizing with her in her impatience of her longer suffering, even virtuously, even piously acquiesce in the recourse to these instruments, which are so sure of destroying the child, and hardly ever fail of doing the mother great and sometimes irreparable mischief.

---

[12] It is among the smaller mischiefs done to the mother, that I here mention my having not unfrequently seen ruptures brought on by the practice of men-midwives, upon patients in other lyings-in, precedently to the one in which I attended them. These ruptures I have sometimes been able to remedy by good management in my laying them.

[13] "Let the *forceps* be unlocked, and the blade *cautiously* disposed under the cloaths, so as not to be *discovered*". Smellie, p. 272.

When then the child has been destroyed, the mother damaged; in satisfaction for all this tragic-work, what have you but perhaps the learned Doctor's assertion, "[14] *that if this force had not been used, the mother must have been lost as well as the child."*

Now granting what is the utmost that candor can be expected to grant, that in but the doubt of the mother's life, it is right to sacrifice the life of the child to that doubt, and much more to the certainty of the mother's life not to be otherwise saved, than by these fatal instruments, I beg and entreat all fathers and mothers, or who are likely to be so, to consider with themselves whether,

In the first place, an experienced midwife is not more likely to prevent such an extremity by previous management, proper anticipations, and actual handiness during the labor-pains, than the aukward man-practitioner (as most of them evidently are) who must, naturally speaking, be so much her inferior in those points of her art, which conduce essentially to the smoothing the way for, and effectuating a delivery; and from the defect of which points that necessity which, is pleaded of a recourse to instruments, originally takes its rise. So that in fact they who are the authors of the danger, pretend to remove it, and how? By an evil inferior to death itself, from which however those are not always safe, to whose safety so much is sacrificed in vain.

In the next place, it may well be recommended to consideration, whether, as the *common methods*[15] confessedly allowed by the men-midwives to be the

---

[14] See Smellie, p. 307.

[15] Smellie, p, 291. "When the head presents, and *cannot* be delivered by the labor-pains; when all the *common methods* have been used without success, the woman being exhausted, and all her efforts vain; and when the child cannot be delivered without such *force* as will *endanger* the *life* of the *mother*, because the head is too large, or the *pelvis* too narrow: it then becomes absolutely necessary to open the head, and extract with the hand, forceps, or crotchet. Indeed this last method formerly was the *common* practice when the child could not be *easily* turned, and is still in use with *those* who do not know how to save the child by delivery with the *forceps*: for this reason their chief care and study was to distinguish, whether the *Fœtus* was dead or alive; and as the *signs* were *uncertain*, the operation was often delayed until the woman was in the most imminent danger; or when it was performed sooner, the operator was frequently accused with *rashness*, on the supposition that the child *might* in time have been delivered *alive* by the *labor-pains*: perhaps he was sometimes conscious to himself, of the *justice* of this *imputation*, although what he had done was with an *upright* intention."— This last indeed would be too uncharitable not to grant.

preferable ones, since the recourse to instruments is not even by them *allowed*, until the *common methods* are exhausted, there is not great reason, without breach of charity, to imagine that the natural unfitness of the men for the *common methods* does not determine especially the common men-midwives to an over-hasty recourse to the *extraordinary* ones, and make them see very *dangerous symptoms*, where they are no better than phantoms of their own creation; so that by their eagerness to embrace them for an excuse, they lose to the patient that benefit of patience in general, which Dr. Smellie himself allows in a particular case[16]. To which patience the midwives are so much more inclined than the men, as indeed they may well be, since, should that even be exhausted, they have no instruments to fly to for the abridgment of a labor: and where they understand their business, not only every thing is best done without them, but the want of them is prevented.

But besides the common motive of impatience in the men-practitioners for resorting to that dangerous expedient of making short work, of which the women are unhappily incapable[17], or at least which the good artists among them hold in the contempt and detestation it deserves; are there no other motives from which recourse may be had to the instruments? I have hinted at some: but as the matter is of infinite importance, from the use made of these instruments, in introducing men into the practice of an art so appropriated to the women, it cannot but be of service even to the public, to discuss the justice

---

[16] Smellie, p. 255. "In this case, we find, *by* experience, that, unless the woman has some VERY DANGEROUS SYMPTOM, the head will in time slide *gradually* down into the *pelvis*, even when it is too *large* to be *extracted* with the *fillet* or *forceps*, and the child be SAFELY delivered by the *labor-pains*, although *slow* and *lingering*, and the mother seems *weak* and *exhausted*, provided she be supported with nourishing and strengthening cordials." Now in this Dr. Smellie is very right; his wrong consists in not making this conclusion more extensive, as that of his fellow-practitioners too often does, in fancying or exaggerating *dangerous symptoms*: whereas for once that nature really occasions them, they are incomparably oftener the effects of the operator's own mis-practice: this observation I cannot, for the truth and importance of it, too often repeat.

[17] In honor to truth, be it here noted, that a few, and very few indeed of the midwives, dazzled with that vogue into which the instruments brought the men, to the supplanting themselves, attempted to employ them, and though certainly they could handle them at least as dexterously as the men, they soon discover'd that they were at once insignificant and dangerous substitutes to their own hands, with which they were sure of conducting their operations both more safely, more effectually, and with less pain to the patient.

at least of some of those hints, and examine whether there is any farther foundation for my fears, that the precipitancy of the men in their resorting to instruments, or to the prematurely forcing a delivery, to the utmost danger if both mother and child, whether, in short, the pretence of extremities may not, in some cases, have even other causes, than a natural incapacity for the *common method*, an ignorance of better practice, or their impatience.

I have before remarked what I here repeat, and repeat it without the least apprehension of being justly taxed with breach of charity, that a mere sordid view of lucre, of supplementing, in short, deficiencies of success in other professions, was originally the foundation in this country of that novel sect of men-midwives, which we have in our days seen so much multiplied. If any can imagine that the instrumentarians, with their crotchets, their forceps, and the rest of their iron or steel apparatus, had more in view the relief of the distressed females, from the dangers to them in the ignorance of the midwives, than they had their own interest, in the stepping into the place of those they so injuriously decried; if any, I say, can believe that sheer humanity, and not sordid gain, was their view, I can only pity a credulity, that must proceed more from a goodness of the heart, than of the head. But to whoever will deign to consult his own reason, exercised upon facts and the nature of things, may easily satisfy himself, that interest, and interest only, inspired and actuated these intruders into a province so little made for them, of which there can hardly be a stronger presumption than the very recommendation of instruments, of which not one of them but must know the perniciousness, though they make it the capital handle of the introduction of themselves. Not one of them but rails at them, and uses them. Now, as I may safely take it for granted, that interest is at the bottom of this innovation, where that same interest is the principle, it will hardly be denied me, that it is generally speaking the leading or the governing one. It is rarely contented with acting a second part. It often exacts sacrifices, but is rarely itself one. All the actions and procedure of its votaries take the tincture of it. Humanity and all the virtuous or tender passions are either totally excluded, or exist with little or no efficacy in a heart enslaved by interest.

In virtue of this reasoning, and I should be much more glad of finding myself mistaken (knowingly I am sure I am not so) than that it should be but too much verified by matter of fact, I shall here submit a case to the reader for his own decision on the probability, and I dare swear, that among the female readers especially, I may chance to have, there will be more than one, who, on her own personal experience, could attest the existence of such a case, or at least has the strongest grounds of presumption of it.

A woman then, lingering in a severe labor, and urged by her pains naturally to wish the speediest end of them, is yet by another superior promptership of nature desirous of meriting the sweet name of mother, and is inclined of herself not to think it over-purchased by a little more patience. In this crisis, much must depend on the judgment, and consequently on the advice of the assistant practitioner, male or female. If a midwife, besides the tenderness constitutional to her sex, her natural fears for the mother especially, not without a due share of concern for the child, where there is a possibility of saving it without too great a risk to the parent, besides the superior execution of her art in points of the manual function, she is moreover bound in all duty to see one labor come to its issue before she undertakes another; for the sake of which, she cannot well, if she would, without instruments, prematurely force a delivery by such violent, dangerous and so often destructive means. She will then in course encourage and inspirit her charge with patience, and use all the blandishments, soothing methods imaginable to comfort, relieve, and strengthen the resolution and spirit of the lying-in-woman. Now, a man-midwife, *well paid*, will perhaps in that cold unaffectionate manner, with which a duty that has no foundation but in interest is ever performed, exhort to endurance that patient whom his dexterity is insufficient to relieve, that patient whose pains are perhaps for the greatest part of his own fault. But should he, during some lingering labor, be called elsewhere, to a more rich employer, or should one from whom he has greater expectations, require an attendance from him incompatible with his duty to his prior employer, is not here a temptation to make a quick dispatch with his instruments? A temptation to which it is at least doubtful whether a man, actuated by interest, may not be over-inclined to yield. It may even byass him, without his perceiving it himself. A man's determining motive, when it is not a very justifiable nature, is often skreened even from himself by a more specious one. Such, in the present case, is the saving the mother, oftenest by destroying, and sometimes by only galling, bruising, or maiming the child, when the mother rarely escapes her share of the suffering. How many mothers have pathetically interceded, and interceded in vain, for a respite of execution, when the operator has in a peremptory tone cut short their instances, by telling them in a magisterial way, that he knew best what to do, and could not answer for the patient's life, if the operation was longer delayed! What reply has a poor woman, weak by nature, oppressed by pain, and subdued by her prepossession to oppose to such an argument of necessity, of which her own life appears to be the favored object? What husband, what friends, but must unhesitatingly subscribe to so just a preference as that of the mother and the child? Not that I would insinuate here, that such a dilemma does not sometimes though certainly very rarely exist: but is it not to be feared, that it is too often rather lightly taken for granted that it does exist? May it not be presumed, that the instruments are brought oftener into use than is necessary, for the sake of a dispatch, of which the child is almost ever the victim, and not unseldom the mother herself, who is always hurt, and sometimes irreparably damaged? May it not be justly suspected, that the abuses of Art have occasioned to many women an appearance of barrenness, from the reality of which kinder Nature had in fact exempted them?

But as if ignorance, inability, impatience, interestedness, were not all of them sufficient motives for the forcing use of these instruments, Dr. Smellie has unmeaningly added another, which alone must, to the greatest number of the men-practitioners, prove a greater excitement than all the others put together, if it be true, that Vanity has so great a predominancy over the human heart as it is generally imagined to have. But let us first quote him: the inference will follow.

"(P. 265.) *at any rate, as* women *are commonly* frightened *at the very name of an* instrument, *it is adviseable to* conceal *them as much as possible,* untill (mind pray that UNTILL) *the* character *of the* operator *is* established.*"

(P. 273.) "*Though the* forceps *are covered with leather, and* appear *so* simple *and* innocent, *I have given directions for* concealing *them, that* young practitioners BEFORE *their* characters *are* fully established, *may avoid the calumnies* and *misrepresentations of those people who are apt to prejudice the ignorant and weak-minded against the use of any instrument, though never so necessary, in this profession; and who taking the advantage of unforeseen accidents which may afterwards happen to the patient, charge the whole misfortune to the* INNOCENT OPERATOR.*"

Here I appeal to every reader of common-sense, to every reader who knows any thing of the human heart, whether it can be imagined that any man-midwife, who is called in to the aid of a lying-in woman, will choose to appear in the character of a *young practitioner*, or of such an one, as that his *character* is not enough *established* to *dare* to use instruments, for fear of after-reflexions. Is not there, if but in this lesson of the Doctor's, couched a strong temptation for a man-practitioner not indeed to produce openly and barefacedly his apparatus of instruments, but to be very uncautious of concealing them? Since the reason for concealing them, that of the women being apt to be frightened at them, stands coupled with another reason, the fittest in the world to work a contrary effect to both; by piquing the vanity of the operator to suffer them to be seen, and what is worse yet, to the using them only that they might be *seen*, especially if to this motive of ostentation you add, that if these instruments the very *grand* and *capital* point of their imaginary *superiority* to the women-practitioners; over whom every occasion of using them seems to the men a kind of triumph.

But while it is to the novices in the art, that Dr. Smellie recommends more especially the concealment of these same terrifying instruments, the good Dr. does not seem aware, that an advice much more honest and humane might be given to the women, for whose *benefit* the instruments are supposed to be invented, which is, not to employ *young practitioners* or novices, not in short to employ those whose character was not *fully* established, since they might, in order to pass for adepts, or at least for no novices, be too apt to embrace occasions of florishing those same instruments with less necessity, if possible, than the *great men* themselves of the profession.

In the mean time, this curious injunction to the *young* practitioners, while the *old* ones are by that distinction implicitly allowed more openness in using the instruments, reminds me of the caution of the Regent-duke of Orleans, who taking monsieur de St. Albin[18], a natural son of his, that was in priest's orders, to task, for some irregularities, of which certain bishops had complained, said to him in their presence, "*Sirrah, could not you stay till you were a bishop?*"

But whatever may be the motives of recourse to instruments, and there are other possible ones which I have omitted, certain it is, that in this nation they

---

[18] At this day archbishop of Cambray.

are more frequently employed than even in France, where that pernicious fashion first took birth. And yet in this very nation it is, that the men-practitioners themselves own, that the less they are used the better. Now will they, to solve this contradiction of their practice to their doctrine, plead that the labors of the women here are, in general, more difficult than they are in France? Common sense and truth will however furnish a juster solution: men-midwives are more employed *here* than in *France*, where the women-practitioners are still respected, and less driven out of practice, consequently instruments are less frequently used. For I will not pay the men-operators of this country so ill a compliment, as to excuse them, by saying they are less dexterous at the manual function than those of France, and therefore the more obliged to have recourse to those instruments, of which they themselves have so ill an opinion, though indeed not a so thoroughly bad one as they deserve.

In the mean while they may well proceed triumphing in their career, notwithstanding all the fatal trips they make in it, while, if they did not even run it in the dark, they have so much learned dust ready to throw into the peoples eyes whom it is so much their interest to blind. No wonder then, that since, in the more severe cases, in the preternatural labors, they so often receive from well-meaning employers both pay and thanks for the greatest mischiefs, owing to their errors both of omission and commission, they should, in the less difficult, and which are by much the most frequent ones, where no tragic accidents have happened, have credit given them for a merit, to which their pretentions are so little examined. For this they are indebted to the overflow of a gratitude at a loss for living object and from an impatience of doubt mistaking that object so grosly, as well as to that same prepossession's continuing, from which they were preferably employed. Hence it is, that one might often hear women, who had not even suffered a little by their practice, from the want of knowing, that by their sincerely say, *"Dr. such an one attended me in my lying-in—He delivered me very well."*—Or, *"I have been lain for four or more children by a man-midwife, and never had room to complain."* All which proves no more than what may very well have happened, that Nature has been too favorable to them, for even the untoward assistance of a man, in the office of a midwife, entirely to frustrate her beneficence. I do not here add the weight that *fashion* throws into the scale of prejudice, reserving to treat of that separately.

But to that conclusion in favor of the men-midwives, from the supposed superiority of their success to that of the women-practitioners, contained in the objection I am now answering, I have further to oppose an argument drawn from *matter of fact*, to which I should imagine it difficult to find a satisfactory reply. This argument then consists in a fair appeal to Experience herself.

I have before observed, that in the Hôtel Dieu at Paris, there are no men-practitioners suffered, for I do not include the surgeon-major, who is absolutely no more than an officer for the form-sake. Consequently there are no instruments ever employed in the delivery of the women admitted to that hospital. It is true they are extremely well taken care of; all necessaries are found them by that noble charity; but yet it cannot be thought, that the same abundance of ease and conveniences can be afforded, as by those persons, generally speaking, who employ men-midwives. This distinction I mention for the sake of the allowance justly to be made in the calculate I am about to propose. Notwithstanding however the superiority in this point on the side of men-midwives practice, notwithstanding the grief of mind from various causes, as well as the bad constitution of the bodies of many of those indigent wretches, prior to the reception into that hospital, notwithstanding other easily conceivable disadvantages; notwithstanding all these, I say, take any given number of patients, delivered purely by the midwives of that hospital, without the intervention of one man-practitioner, and especially without instruments, and to that given number, oppose an equal one of women attended from the first of their labor to their delivery by the men-midwives, and see on the fide of which sex, in the operators, there will be found the greater number of those who shall have done well, or suffered least.

I am the more emboldened to propose such an experiment from my own certain knowledge. I have seen more than two thousand women delivered under my eyes, at the Hôtel-Dieu at Paris, some of whose cases must be readily imagined to have been severe or preternatural ones. Yet all of them were delivered by our midwives and apprentices without the aid of a man-practitioner; nor an instrument so much as thought of. And in all this number I can safely aver, there were but four who died upon their lying-in; and that not from any fault of the midwife's art; but one from the complication of a dropsy, the other three, who were daughters to honest tradesmen, sunk under the shock of grief and shame at the being deserted by the men who had brought them into that condition. They died, in short, of their desire to die. Yet the children all did well.

This is a fact that does not require the being believed upon my word. The known practice at that hospital, and the registers regularly kept, will attest the truth of this computation. And here, I appeal to every intelligent reader's own sense, to his own knowledge of things, whether it is unfairly presumed, that in the same number of two thousand women, delivered by the men-practitioners, they could show a roll so innocent, so free from fatal mischief or damage to their patients, to mother and to child. Let any parents, or who may hope to be parents, or are concerned but for the interest of mankind in population, weigh but the force of this argument, purely drawn from a matter of fact, of which there can be so few who are not, in some measures, judges enough to decide upon their own knowledge, or at least on strong grounds or belief or conjecture. In such a number as two thousand women delivered by the men-operators, how many, by what I know, and by what many others must know as well as I, must have perished, or been torn, ruptured, grievously hurt, or irreparably damaged! How many innocent infants must have lost their little lives, in proof of that superiority of practice in the men to the women! Or rather, in proof of that infatuate credulity, which has prevailed in favour of an innovation so unauthorized by nature, by common sense, or by experience!

OBJECTION THE THIRTEENTH.

Say what you will, the fashion will predominate. It is now the fashion to prefer men-practitioners of midwifery to midwives. You will oppose the torrent in vain.

ANSWER.

The conclusion against me that I shall oppose the torrent in vain, is a very just one. As to myself, I ought to expect that, I should oppose it in vain, if the decision of the public was to turn upon any thing of so little authority as my private opinion, especially in a point where it is so justly liable to the suspicion of its being byassed, both by private interest, and partiality to my own sex. I readily then grant that my own opinion should go for nothing. But what ought to go for a great deal is my reader's own judgment, formed upon his own reason and knowledge. But that is not all. I have some dependence on Nature and common sense recovering their rights, from this preference of the men-midwives which shocks both, being, in truth, nothing more than a fashion, not even of the growth of this country, but transplanted from a neighbouring one, whose follies are unhappily so contagious, though for the most part so despicable. How a few interested men, for want of business in their own professions, transplanted this baneful exotic here, where it has met with such undue cherishment has already been touched upon.

But then as this unnatural preference has all the folly and whim of fashion in it, it may be hoped, that it will also have all the instability and transitoriness of one. Time that confirms the dictates of Nature destroys the fictions of opinion. But in points where Nature is herself attacked or injured, inconveniencies and damages never fail of following thereon, enough to oppose duration of them. The numbers of lying-in women (thanks to beneficent Nature) rather not destroyed than duly assisted by the men-operators, can neither atone for those who perish, sometimes the mother, sometimes the child, sometimes both, while none of them are but sufferers in some degree; nor long blind a public, that has so much interest not to be imposed upon in a matter so essential to it, by false pretences, or by an injurious and interested degradation of the midwives, who at the worst can hardly be so bad as the very best of the men, in the capital point of their business, the manual function. The oftenest greater *danger*, and always the greater *pain*, under men-operators than under the midwives hands will, sooner or later, determine the parties concerned to open their eyes on their greatest interest, in a point of such infinite importance to them.

Granting then to Fashion all the power it really has, and a greater one it is, than for the honor of human kind, can well be imagined, still, it not only has its limits of extension, but duration. It is only for the truth of Nature to be universal and eternal.

Fashion, it is true, may not only govern people in indifferent matters, such as dress, furniture, equipage, or so forth, but even in essential, even in capital ones, such, for example, as is this point of option between the men-operators and the midwives: it may, in short, exert its tyranny in many things, one would rather think left better to the determination of REASON. But then this tyranny cannot well be long-lived. The evils which such a fashion begets destroy at length their own parent. No opinion then, as I have before observed, can be permanent that is not founded on the truth of Nature: but where the consequences of such an opinion are detrimental to the good of society, which is the darling object of Nature; that spirit of self-preservation which she has so manifestly diffused thro' human kind, will hardly suffer errors pernicious to it long to subsist. There is no fashion can, under such objections, long hold out against victorious Nature, who is sure to revenge the violences offered her.

And here I even officiously seize on an occasion that rises to me out of the very bowels, I may say, of my subject, of selecting for one proof of the danger of adopting innovations offensive to Nature, a point of such near analogy to midwifery, as that of nursing children, the care of whom, next to that of the mothers, is the true midwife's tender province.

I wish then that those, who too readily admit that this so recent a fashion of employing men-midwives preferable to female ones, is an improvement receivable on the foot of its supposed advantage to human kind, would consider a little the actual consequences of having flown in the face of Nature with respect to the bringing up young children, in a way scarce more foreign from her dictates, than that of *men* delivering *women*. That women are by Nature herself formed for the office of aiding women in their lying-in; that they are also formed to bring up children by the breast, are two parts of their destination by Nature, which in all ages, in all countries seem to have born little or no controversy. Interest has lately invaded both these provinces. With this difference, that as to the first, that of women supplanted in their business of delivering women, an active interest has prevailed; as in that of denying the female breast to children, it is a purely passive one[19]; and we shall soon see what a dreadful effect this sacrifice of Nature to interest has produced.

---

[19] By this interest, with respect to the mis-government of the infants that fall upon the parish, I do not mean such a personal interest, as that the super-intendants of the charity put a single farthing into their own private pockets, out of the savings, by the with-holding or grudging a proper provision for the children, but merely the interest of a parish, or the public, in so false and inhuman an article of parcimony. A consideration which, if that were possible, renders it the more inexcusable from the temptation being so much the less.

As to the mischief produced by the other, of the implicitly excluding the women from midwifery, by the power of prejudice and fashion, it is not, as yet, of a Nature for obvious reasons quite so susceptible of proof, though most certainly not the less therefore existent. And that mischief is palpably owing to the gain which the men-midwives find or presume in the exercise of that profession. This is the active interest: that end to which the means give so justly the construction of base and sordid. The rich are the object of this wretched imposition, which will probably last so much the longer, for the interest to be found in imposing upon them.

But for the denying the female breast to children; it has not indeed passed hitherto into a tenet, that children may as well be reared by the spoon as by the breast, because there is not that prospect of the place of a *dry-nurse* being as lucrative as that of a *man-midwife*. If it was so, I should not dispair of seeing a great he-fellow florishing a pap-spoon as well as a forceps, or of the public being enlightened by learned tracts and disputations, stuffed full of Greek and Latin technical terms, to prove, that water-gruel or scotch-porridge was a much more healthy aliment for new-born infants than the milk of the female breast, and that is was safer for a man to dandle a baby than for an insignificant woman.

As this unnatural treatment then of children is almost entirely as yet confined to the very poor, that is to say, to new-born babes thrown upon the public CHARITY for their SUSTENANCE, the rearing by the spoon is not yet regularly established as a general *doctrine*, it is only admitted in PRACTICE! As *proper* wet-nurses, from the difficulty in procuring them, might be *dearer* than dry ones; the *cheapest* method is preferred, and forms a kind of passive interest or saving œconomy.

But what are the consequences of this violation of Nature, in the grudging her peculiarly appointed aliment to these poor little candidates for life? What follows the substituting, for cheapness-sake, such food as is meant to be afforded them, and is perhaps sometimes even not given them? Death. Death with all that cruelty of torture that attends atrophy or inanition. Thus perish these miserable victims to the false opinion, that the course of Nature can be changed with impunity. I have said here false opinion only, because, with all the obduracy of heart that the spirit of interest so notoriously creates, with all the crimes it so often produces, I cannot think, that such an horror, as the

88

murder of so many innocents, can be entirely imputed to interest without ignorance coming in for its share, though interest has doubtless contributed to the so long continuance of it.

If that maxim is not a false one, that he who knowingly suffers an innocent person to perish, and can help it, is actually guilty of murder: and I prefer here the term of guilty to that of accessary; because I am told, that where there is guilt of murder, all are in the eye of equity and law, principals. Ignorance then, of the sure murder of these innocents by their method of treatment, can be the only plea for those to whom the national charity had committed the care of them. I should think too, that even I myself sinned against charity, if I did not believe, that there is none of those trustees of poor children, that would not shudder at the thought, of himself taking an infant up by the leg and dashing its brains out against the wall. And yet that would be balmy mercy, the dispatch considered, compared to the lingering tortures, in which those poor little creatures must expire, in the common way of parish-nursing. What is certain however is, that Death would scarce more assuredly be the consequence of the child's brains being at once beat out, than of that impropriety of aliment, which in the mildest construction is owing to an error in opinion or belief, than any aliment could be salutarily substituted to the one dictated by Nature.

I have here mentioned barely impropriety, or sometimes negation of aliment, without allowance for other causes of destruction to those infants, such as cold, bad air, uncleanliness, neglect of due attendance, or deficiency, in short, of requisites, which are not to be expected from the very poorer sort of the people, to whom the rearing of those infants is generally committed. But that omission of mine is neither undesigned nor unfair. I presume I shall have the greatest physicians on my side, in averring, that even new-born babes are endowed with a surprizing hardiness. Their little seemingly so delicate bodies bear cold to a degree scarcely credible, but from the commonness of both observation and practice, that they only thrive the better for immersions in cold water. Cleanliness, a good air, and attendance, have doubtless indeed some share in the well-doing of children of that age: but all together are in no degree of comparison to the importance of bestowing on children their appropriate aliment. The physical disquisitions into the reason of this do not belong to me here: nor are a few instances of infants reared by the spoon any valid justification for breaking the general rule of Nature, assigning to the female breast the nutrition of children: of which too there is salutary consequence, that in the very act of lactation there is, by Nature, generated such an indearment of the suckled child to the nurse[20], as that she who began it perhaps only for hire, finds herself engaged by a growing affection to supply in some measure the place of the mother to the orphan or deserted babe. The rearing by the spoon is so far from inspiring any such dearness, that the innocent infant is considered only as an imbarassment, of which the quicker the riddance, in the death of the *brat*, so much the better.

The opinion, however, that this one of the greatest institutes of Nature for the preservation of the species, for which she has so admirably organized the female breast, could be dispensed with in favor of a most sordid savingness, has alone caused more human sacrifices, to that black Demon of INTEREST, than probably were ever made to the "grim idol of" Moloch in the valley of Hinnom, while the cries of the poor children could not be heard by ears closely stopped up in honor of that infernal spirit.

But if any reader should imagine that I here invent any thing, or that, in favor of my inference of danger from the case of revolting against the unalterable institutes of Nature, I have exaggerated matters, nothing will be more easy, nor probably at the same more shocking, than the procuring himself a proof of the scarce not actual murders I have mentioned.

The parish-registers of this great metropolis are, I presume, open for inspection. There needs but to examine them, to discover the red-letter catalogue of the armies of innocents that have been put to death under the management of the charity destined to preserve their life. There will be found not one but many, even of the most populous parishes, where for fourteen, twenty, or more years, not one poor babe of the thousands taken in have escaped the general destruction, and sacrifice to the inhuman fiend of Hell, *Interest*. Here with what propriety might Nature borrow from one of her most dutiful children and darling, the following exclamation,

---

[20] I have somewhere read, that brutes have not been insensible of this effect, on suckling animals, though even of so different a kind from their own, that the most mortal enmity naturally existed between them: such was the instance, transmitted from Pennsylvania, of a cat so softened towards a rat, by having accidentally given suck to it amongst its own kittens, that it forbore exerting towards it its usual hostility to that species.

———— ———— ALL my pretty ones?
Did you say ALL! what ALL?
I cannot but remember such things were,
That were most PRECIOUS to me: did Heav'n look on,
And would not take their part? ACCURSED INTEREST,
They were all STRUCK for thee!

This is so rigidly true of some parishes, that if I am not misinformed, the verification was not long ago made, as to one of them before a court of justice, of not a single infant having been brought up in the term of fourteen years. And I could name another, in which, during the course of above twenty years, ALL, ALL the new-born children that fell under the administration of the Parish-CHARITY, perished, except one boy, of whom it is recorded as a prodigy, that he lived till he was five years of age, when he filled up the number, and died like the rest. Will any one here say, that the total mortality was purely accidental?

But this can be now wonder to those who know there is such an expression, even proverbially in use, as that of children being a BURTHEN to the parish. An expression of which it is hard to pronounce whether it is more execrable or more silly. But what is so inconsequential as the spirit, or rather the no-spirit of interest? Children may indeed be a burthen to private families; and yet for the sweetness of it, how cheerfully is it oftenest born, or with very few extraordinary exceptions to the general rule? But to a nation, or what is the same thing, to the lawful representative of the nation, a parish, what can be on earth a falser light to view children in, than that of a burthen? What could be so intolerable in the sum to be added to that actually paid for their being worse than murdered out of hand, to save their little lives, and bring them up to that age, in which the national wisdom should have established for them, at once, the means of earning their likelihood, and of earning it with such beneficial retribution to their truly mother-country, as should amply reward her for her not having neglected the duties of humanity towards them? All the good, all the sensible part of mankind allow, that the true riches of a state, are in the numerousness of its subjects. Trade, arts, the navy, the militia, our colonies all open inexhaustible channels of employment and maintenance. And yet there are who can call children, those children too of the public, not in a ludicrous, but in the dearest tenderest sense, since in the public they ought to find that

91

office of a parent, of which the guilt, the inability, the want of nature in their natural relations, or their death may have defrauded them; there are, I say, who can call such children a *burthen*! We complain of the defect of population, and yet have seen interest creative of obduracy, and perpetuating ignorance and error, manifestly thinning the species, by nipping those tender blossoms of human kind.

Here, if this notice of the treatment of children should even appear a digression, I should, in favor of the intention, hope forgiveness from a humane reader. He would scarce impute it to me as matter for criticism, the having sacrificed propriety to the introduction of a point so important to humanity. But the truth is, that neither as a digression, nor as a false or overstrained argument, nor as a misapplication, can the same well be considered, by any who will withal consider its strict affinity in so many points to the subject of which I am treating.

It will readily appear, that both these violences offered to Nature in the substituting the men-midwives to the females, and dry-nurses to wet-ones, acknowledge exactly the same common parent, interest, and have exactly the same common effect, the destruction of infants. Is it then possible to be too much on one's guard against those so flagrant impositions, which are the offspring of that proof-hardened passion? Is any thing sacred from it, since the lives of innocents palpably have not been so, in one branch of practice, nor very presumably are on jot more respected in the other? It is true indeed, that the practice of employing dry-nurses has not yet ascended much among the great and rich; first, because fashions rarely do ascend from the lower classes of life, and next, because there is no such temptation of actual lucre to defend or spread it: but as to that of preferring men-midwives, nothing is so likely as its descending, as it is so much the nature of fashion to descend, and none are more readily adopted by the lower ranks of people from the higher ones, than those fashions which are the most foolish and the most pernicious. And certainly this is not the one that the least deserves those epithets.

Was it not for this influence of the fashion, in making the most unreasonable as well as the most dangerous things pass into practice from the highest down to the lowest life, many an honest man might escape the bad consequences of his following the example of those, than whom none are so liable to be imposed on in such matters, the great and the opulent. These make it worth the while of interested persons to deceive them, and thus often for being cheated, pay with their money, their health, and even with their lives. In the mean time, many who are seduced by the vogue in which they see the men-midwives, employ them on a principle which cannot be enough commended, their natural affection to their wives and children. The reasoning which occurs to a husband in middling or low life on this occasion is probably as follows. "My wife and child are full as dear to me as those of the greatest man in the kingdom are to him, and shall I grudge a little more expence in the provision for their greater *safety*?" So far he reasons right: all his mistake lies in taking too readily for granted, that same *greater safety*, to be on the side of the men-practitioners in preference to the midwives, because the former are employed by the great, who, by the by, consult Nature the least of any class of life, even in points of their own health. And certainly in many respects to that *sine-quo-non* of human happiness, the great had better follow the example even the poor, than the poor theirs. Make the most then of your reasoning from the prevalence of fashion, the gout and the men-midwives, well considered, are no very enviable appendixes of high-life.

If in some that laudable tenderness for mother and child, is the determining consideration for employing a man-midwife by whom Nature, if consulted, would assure all concerned, that the safety of both was more likely to be endangered than not, there are others again, in whom calling in the aid of a man-midwife is rather matter of luxury, of parade or ostentation, than of opinion of superiority safety. These are of that imitative kind of beings, with whom the preference of a man-practitioner for the conducting of his wife's lying-in, turns upon no other motive, than what would equally make them bestow a silk gown of a new fashion, or a laced-head upon her; from a spirit of emulation of some neighbour or superior.

But what is more surprising yet, is that notwithstanding the kind of loathing and repugnance with which Nature inspires the women to receive such an office from a man, as that of delivering them, a repugnance to which they had so much better listen, since it has all the characters of a salutary instinct; there are women so weak, as not only not to represent to their husbands the expedience of examining, at least, the propriety of such a fashion, before they blindly adopt it on the faith either of others liable to be deceived, or of those interested in the deceiving them; but who even, in a ridiculous complaisance to that fashion, of which themselves and children are not unlikely to be the victims, will make a point of being attended by a man-midwife, by way of a piece of state.

I have myself known women so infected by this silly vanity, that on receiving visits from their friends after lying-in, and being delivered by a woman, with the utmost safety and satisfaction to them, have been ashamed of having had the better sense and regard for themselves, to employ a midwife in defiance of the fashion, and have told their friends, that it is true Mrs. —— had lain them, but that there was a Doctor at hand in the next room. This by the by was false, for such a *Led-Doctor* is neither needed nor employed, where a midwife that knows her business is called. If any occasion for medical or even chirurgical skill arises from the complication of a case, there is always time to have the advice of a regular physician, or a regular surgeon, because that complication can never escape timely notice. It can only then be, for the sake of his iron and steel instruments, that a man-midwife has so much as the pretext of being necessary, and I hope to prove, that all the needful can be much better done without them. Yes, I repeat it, better done without them.

For here and throughout the reader will please to observe, that it is on the superiority of safety in employing midwives that I impugn the growing fashion of a recourse to men-practitioners. It is the side of Nature I take against a set of mean mercenaries, who commit the cruellest outrages upon her, under the falsest of all pretences in them, that of assisting her. I would not be so criminal as to wish the benefit of a false argument, in a point of life and death to those mothers and children, my tender care, even could I be silly enough to imagine; that I could pass such an one upon my reader. I wave therefore all plea of the novelty of this upstart profession of men-midwives. Such a plea I readily confess is not receivable. Were it so, how many valuable discoveries or improvements must have been stifled in their birth, if the objection to their being novelties was a valid one? All that I would contend for is, that an innovation should not be admitted only because it is an innovation; and that the decision of a matter of such capital importance, is better left to Reason, always herself submissive to Nature, than abandoned to Fashion, which so often acknowledges no other jurisdiction than that of whim or humor.

There is no prescription for error, no sanction in custom against improvements. But certainly in such a capital point as the life of so many human creatures, in short, in one of the most sacred objects of government, that of population, such a novelty as that of bringing men-midwives into general practice, requires rather a greater authority than that of Fashion, while there is such a standard of essay as Reason.

Inoculation was not long since a novelty in this nation. The lady who introduced it, for any thing I know to the contrary, still lives to enjoy the honor of having procured so great a benefit to mankind. But then this benefit would bear the fairest of all trials, that of calculation: for what is reason itself but another word for calculation? The procuring then the small-pox by inoculation, in a body duly prepared, and especially at an eligible age, affords, according to the doctrine of chances, so much a fairer prospect of safety, than in the case of a spontaneous or accidental infection, that nothing scarcely could be imagined more friendly to Nature than such a rational prevention of her danger, from a distemper too rarely escaped, for the possibility of that escape to be employed as an argument against such a method of prevention. Here then the seeming violence offered to Nature, appeals for its justification to Nature, Reason and Experience.

Consult Nature as to this innovation in the employing men-practitioners preferably to the midwives, who have been for ages, and so universally considered as the properest for that function. Nature will tell you, that it is injuring her to suspect her of being so cruel a mother-in-law, as to deny her tenderest production the female sex sufficient succors within herself, or leave women under a necessity of recurring to men for aid in their greatest need of it, during those sufferings, to which it has pleased the great master of Nature to subject peculiarly the women. If Nature then is but another name for his Fiat through all his works, never was his will more plainly signified than by her voice in this point: a repugnance in both sexes to that office being administered by a man. A repugnance which is not even one of Nature's least remarkable signs of abhorrence from this innovation, and is only to be surmounted in the men by interest, and in the women by their false fear, or what is weaker yet, by their rage in following that bell-weather Fashion, though it should lead them like sheep to the slaughter. The uncouthness and inaptitude of the men, so ill compensated by their miserable inventions of iron and steel instruments, form another loud protest of Nature against this important function being committed to men-operators.

Consult reason, and reason founded upon those dictates of Nature, to which time only gives the more strength, will tell you, in contempt of fashion, that the men-midwives will never do any thing in a matter rather too universal for any excellence in it to depend upon Greek, Latin, or Arabic; that they are, in short, only hatching of wind-eggs, in the study of an art, which no incubation on it will ever sufficiently naturalize to them.

If to experience you appeal, I have already furnished unrefutable arguments of that's being against the men-midwives. But let them remember my confession, that the number which I have quoted of women happily delivered is taken from the course of practice of good midwives. I am not here an advocate for bad ones, nor would I wish to authorize them if I could. All that I shall say, and dare aver is, that the very worst of them, unless their hands are cut off, or at least deserve to be cut off, can hardly be worse than the best of the men-operators.

But while it is to the tribunal of Nature, of Reason, and of Experience, that I presume to wish that this same Fashion might be brought; I readily acknowledge its force though not its justice. I feel the power of it, with pain, for the sake of humanity[21]! My opposition then to this fashion is rather founded in duty than in hope. The weakness of it will probably furnish only a new matter of triumph, not indeed over me who am too low for it, but over the welfare of mankind, which it has often, in more points than this, the pleasure to see sacrificed to it, though in not one perhaps more palpably than in this one.

In the mean time it might be worth the while of even those who not being themselves men-midwives, nor having any personal interest in patronizing them, owe their favorable notion of them to their own fair judgment; it would, I say, even be worth their while to consider that there may possibly be

---

[21] The candid reader will please to observe, that in giving up so much as I do of the argument from the prevalence of fashion, I do not give up a little: since I might justly oppose to it the instances of our Royal Family, in which we see so many happily living and florishing monuments of the midwives' capacity. *Accoucheurs* had, I presume, no *hand* in delivering the greatest Lady in this kingdom. The men-midwives will perhaps treat this as trifling. But what will they say to so victorious a proof in favor of the female-practitioners, as that taken from themselves, who, for the most part, were obliged to the midwives for their ushering them into that world, of which they are so much the light and ornament; and out of which world they are rather not so gratefully employed in driving those, by whose function they were helped into it?

a time, when they may themselves see reason to change that judgment of theirs. They may possibly discover the illusions of interest, under the old stale mask of service to the public. They may find out the folly of fashion. But will not it be too late, when that fury of fashion shall, like a pestilence, have either swept away the good midwives, or at least have so thinned their numbers, as not to leave enough for the demand of the service? They must in time become, to all intents and purposes, like an old obsolete law, as effectually abolished by disuse, as if abrogated by a formal repeal. "The matter would not be much if they were," an instrumentarian will probably say, but I doubt much, whatever he might gain by it, whether mankind or population would profit much by that extermination, even though the men-midwives with their tire-têtes, crotchets, and forceps, were to succeed to their business.

And that such an extermination is far from improbable, will appear no strained inference to those who consider the power of Fashion, which establishes its tyranny, much as the first Roman emperors did theirs over that commonwealth, by leaving a semblance of liberty without the substance; whence the baneful effects do not the less follow, or rather the more surely follow. Thus there is indeed as yet no act of parliament for the preference of men-practitioners or the extinction of the midwives, but the statutes of fashion are not only more forcible than any act of a human legislature, but, in this matter even than the laws of Nature herself tho' inculcating their observance, under pain of death, or at least of severe corporal punishment; such as being torn with cold pinchers, or cut or punctured with instruments, or put to more pain than necessary.

Already has fashion driven numbers of women out of their livelihood to make way for the encroachments of the men on the female provinces of industry, though there never was a time, in which it was not a just complaint that there were rather much too few means of employment for women. Fashion has determined it otherwise, and many callings formerly appropriated to females are now exercised by men.

But as to this profession of midwifery, even the total extinction of the real midwives, would not be perhaps so bad as giving that name to those poor to those poor creatures in training under the men-practitioners, who independently of their own incapacity of practice, consequently of forming good practitioners, have a palpable interest not to suffer their women-pupils to gain any eminence in the profession that might give umbrage to themselves[22]. The midwives whom these men-practitioners would perhaps gratiously allow to subsist, might to their own insufficiency add the dangerous circumstance of creating, or at least of not preventing, by duly exerting themselves in the pre-disposing part, the necessity of calling in their protectors, especially where recommended by them. Not that I imagine even these mock-midwives would willfully be guilty of such prevarication in their duty. For them not to deserve such a suspicion, it is enough that they are women, consequently tender-hearted. But that does not exclude the idea of weakness. But where so fair a virtue as gratitude may disguise even themselves the fouler motive of interest lurking at bottom, if that tenderness is not even destroyed, it may not impossibly be made a tool of, and join in persuading them, that things had really better be left to the men-practitioners, whose creatures are devotees they are. Thence a negligence superadded to their defect of skill. Such subalterns then would, at least, not be dis-inclined to the "FINDING" *themselves* "AT A LOSS", or yet worse for the patient, have by their omissions, if not commissions, bred the occasion of *"finding"* themselves *"at that loss"*, even mechanically, and without the direct design of paying their court to their recommending *"accoucheur, their man of honor and real friend,"* in a *candid* recourse to him. Pity it were indeed that so charming a harmony should not subsist between *the accoucheurs* and such *midwives*, for

---

[22] Pray remark the following directions for the *choice* of a midwife, from Dr. Smellie, p. 448.

"She (the midwife) ought to *avoid* ALL *reflections* upon *men-practitioners*, and when she finds herself *at a loss*, candidly have recourse to their assistance: on the other hand, this *confidence* ought to be *encouraged* by the *men*, who, when called, instead of openly condemning her method of practice (even though it should be *erroneous*) ought to make allowance for the weakness of the sex, and rectify what is amiss, without exposing her mistakes. This conduct will as effectually conduce to the welfare of the patient, and operate as a silent rebuke upon the conviction of the midwife, who, finding herself treated so tenderly, will be more *apt* to *call* necessary assistance on future occasions, and to consider the ACCOUCHEUR as a MAN OF HONOR and a REAL FRIEND. These gentle methods will prevent that calumny, which too often prevail among the male and female practitioners; and redound to the ADVANTAGE of both: for no ACCOUCHEUR is so *perfect*, but that he may err sometimes, and on such occasions he must expect to meet with retaliations from those midwives whom he may have roughly used."

the "MUTUAL ADVANTAGE" of both! A harmony, which however could hardly be established but at the expence of the sacrificed patients.

And here I appeal to the reader's own fair judgment, whether I over-strain the consequence against such wretched creatures as they cannot but be who must, for bread, be so subservient to the men-midwives, and be what the French call, their *ames damnées* (souls sold). Can any thing be more probable than that these *good women* dignified by the men-practitioners, out of their special grace and favor with the title of midwives, will on all occasion consult the "*advantage*" of their kind *patrons* and "*real friends*". And how can that advantage be better consulted than by bungling their work so as to make it *appear* necessary to have a candid recourse to the good Doctor, who recommended and warranted them? can it, in short, be imagined, that they will be less mere machines than Dr. Smellie's Dolls, or indeed furnish less occasion, than the education under those Dolls, for the *iron* and *steel instruments*, which are the most part understood to be indispensably necessary where the midwife shall have failed. And as to such midwives as have been formed or recommended by the men-practitioners, their *not* failing would indeed be the wonder!

Thus the name of a midwife may subsist after the reality shall have perished, and the world so often deceived by mere names, may not perhaps discover this annihilation till long after it is effectuated, or till it is too late to repair the damages, which will hardly fail of discovering it to them. Of good midwives there never were too many; but they are now much too few; though still not more rare in proportion than those of the men-midwives, who may be called good, comparatively to so many of them as are dangerously superficial. Discouragement has already greatly hindered the places of the good female-practitioners who are gone off the stage, from being duly supplied. Proper subjects decline taking up a profession, in which they must have to dread the prevalence of so false a prejudice against them, as that which determines the preference of the male-operators. It is easier to destroy, than to create a-new; and perhaps when the need of good midwives shall be at the greatest, the difficulty of finding such, will make the employing of men-practitioners, with all the so just objections to them, even a necessity. Things are not at present perhaps far from that point, and an alarming consideration that would be to all women, if they were but to reflect on the increase of pain and danger to themselves in the hours already too big with both, of their increase, I say, by the most aukward and violent aid of the men, compared to the so much more effectual and gentle methods so natural to the women-assistants.

If the parties then principally concerned in the decision of this question, and especially the women who are the patients, and their tender relations of husband, father, or brother, &c. were but to consult their own feelings, their reason, and even that instinct which, in this point, is itself so strong a reason from its being the voice of Nature never unhearkened to with impunity, they would soon, to your objection drawn from a fashion scarce less ridiculous than pernicious, allow no more weight than, in fact, it deserves.

OBJECTION THE FOURTEENTH.

You must allow, however, that it must be a false modesty that, in the women, which can oppose the preference of the men-practitioners to the female ones.

ANSWER.

I know indeed that Dr. Smellie (page 2. of his introduction) attributes the opposition made by the Athenian women[23] to the prohibition of midwives,

---

[23] As the story is told in Hyginus, it should seem that the practice of midwifery at Athens, was, on a season interdicted to the women, who, by a fixt resolution to die rather than submit to be delivered by the men, procured from the Areopagus the repeal of that statute, and the saving from imminent condemnation one Agnodice, who had dressed herself in mens cloaths, to elude the cognizance of the law. The great practice she had obtained by this means had alarmed the physicians, who thereon accused her as a seducer of the women: against which she easily defended herself by a declaration of her sex. But this brought her under the penalty of the law against women exercising the midwife's profession. The story imperfectly related in Hyginus, at the same time that it does honor to the modesty of the Athenian women, that is to say, if modesty is not, according to the men-midwives, a false honor, gives room to suspect, that the midwives themselves had perhaps occasioned the promulgation of so absurd a law. It is well known, than in those antient times, there were for female disorders women-physicians in form. Perhaps their encroachments on the province of the men, by exercising the art of physic in general, might make a restraint necessary, which was only so far faulty as that the remedy was in this, as it often is in other cases, carried into extremes. I would no more

and to the acceptance of men-practitioners in their room to "*mistaken modesty.*" It may however with more reason and truth be averred, that the admittance of men to that function by women, would be in the women a most egregiously MISTAKEN IMMODESTY. Since, surely the virtue or grace of female modesty is not an object to be held so cheap, as to be sacrificed for worse than nothing, for nothing better, in short, than the purchase with it of danger or perdition to both the mother and child. After so valuable a sacrifice as that of a modesty itself, it may perhaps sound mean to add any thing comparatively, so trifling as that of the hire not given to the person who prostitutes herself in some sort on a so much mistaken hope, but to the very person to whom she is prostituted in that hope of superior safety.

I am not then here to assume a character, that would become me so ill, of a Casuist or Divine, by pretending to fix the degree of moral turpitude in the submission of modest women to a practice, which, I will even allow might be justified by the superior consideration of safety to two lives, if that consideration was not a question most impudently begged, with so little foundation, that the very contrary thereof is the truth.

Neither would I here incur the just charge of impertinence, in giving my private and insignificant opinion on an undecency so unwarranted by any necessity. That would look too like dictating to others, what they are to think of a practice, of which every one will doubtless judge for himself. The boundaries of female modesty are so well known, and so ascertained by common consent, that surely it little belongs to me to offer new lights upon that subject.

What I have then to say, on this head, is purely in justification of that modesty, which the men-midwives are for obvious reasons pleased to call a false one, though so far as it pleads for excluding them, it is an ingratitude to that Nature, of which it is the peculiar gift to the female sex, not to term it even a wise virtue.

Society especially stands indebted to Nature for her suggestion of modesty in this point. If in all ages, in all civilized countries, the wife is considered as the peculiar property of a husband, insomuch, that all laws human and divine

---

justify the women overstepping their proper sphere of employment into that of the men, than I would the men sinking into that of women. They are both reprehensible, both dangerous, but assuredly, the last must be the most ridiculous.

consecrate, if I may use the expression, to him alone, exclusive of all other men, the access to the reserved parts of the wife's body, certainly such a privilege can hardly be thought lightly communicable. And what can be more so than suffering a man, mercenarily or wantonly, or perhaps both, to invade that so sacred property, under the mask of a service, for which he is by Nature so evidently disqualified? While Nature too has made so ample a provision for this very service, in fitting the women for it, with so much more propriety and safety, both to the concern of the public in the welfare of population, as well as to the domestic honor of families, which is not without some danger, at least, from the practice of midwifery being in the hands of men.

As to this last averment of mine, the truth of it is so glaring, that it does not even need Dr. Smellie's own implicit confession of it, in his instructions to the men-practitioners in general, or, if you please, to his more than nine hundred pupils.

"He (the ACCOUCHEUR*) ought to* ACT *and* SPEAK *with the utmost* DELICACY *of* DECORUM, *and* NEVER VIOLATE *the* TRUST *reposed in him, so as to harbor the least* IMMORAL *or* INDECENT *design; but demean himself in all respects suitable to the* DIGNITY *of his* PROFESSION," p. 447.

Here I confess myself so smitten with the propriety and sanctity of the precept of the good Doctor's, and particularly with the needfulness of it, that I would advise every man-practitioner of midwifery, of a certain age that might require it, to have said commandment wrote out in *gold letters*, and wear it about his arm, especially on his proceeding to *officiate*, by way of amulet, phylactery or preservative against any incident temptation to *violate* his *trust*, or to fall off from the high *dignity* of his profession. All that I fear is, that its virtue may not always be to be depended upon, against the energy planted by nature in the difference of the sexes. No one would be farther than I from the cruel injustice of drawing consequences unfavorable to any set of men, from the misconduct of any particular individual in it. [24]Errors are

---

[24] It is from this principle, that, with so fair a field for raillery, often not the least forcible of arguments, I have, against those who are such advocates for the use of *anatomy* in *midwifery*, abstained from laying any stress on the famous imposition of the Rabbet-woman of Godalmin, upon professors of anatomy. I am so far from attacking anatomy, that I aver, every good midwife ought to know *enough* of it to assist her practice. This would not however constitute her an anatomist, nor is it requisite that she should be one.

purely personal. If I then so much as mention the case of a man-midwife convicted of having debauched a gentleman's wife, in consequence of his admission to the practice of his profession of midwifery upon her, it is by no means neither with a design to insult the unhappy criminals, nor to draw from thence an inference to the disfavor of the men-practitioners in this point, beyond what I am authorized by the constancy of the temptation from Nature, to all, yes, to all, who, by their age, in one sex, are not past it: I say in one sex, because in the other, the female, the very circumstances of a woman's needing a midwife, shews that she is not past the age of, at least, causing a temptation. Further, it would even be a matter of argument on the side of the men-midwives, that so *few* instances come to the knowledge of the public, of the ill-consequence of a practice which breaks down the capital barriers of modesty; if those ill-consequences were not, in the nature of them, not only a secret, but easy to be kept secret. Who would complain but the husband or relations of transactions between a man-midwife and his patient? But then how seldom need a third to be let into such a secret?

I would not then have the men-midwives to be too forward to treat the modesty of the women on this head as a false one, or their scruples as a weakness. Modesty in this case is not only the safeguard of the lives of themselves and children, but of their own honor, which if it does not receive an actual fall in such a subjection to a man-midwife, had perhaps better not be so unnecessarily risked so near the brink of the precipice.

I am not writing here for Italians or Spaniards, or any of the inhabitants of those countries who are so prone to jealousy, perhaps because they know their women. I am now addressing myself to Englishmen, not jealous, because, if they know theirs, they must know that, in proportion to the number, no women on the earth have more of the reality of virtue and modesty. I will not suppose then any thing so offensive, as that the chastity of the generality of them is not infinitely superior to the advantages or overtures for design afforded the men admitted to such a privacy, as that of attending them in their lying-in and delivering them. But would the honestest woman, or one however sure of herself or of her virtue, think it eligible, without a full satisfactory proof of that superior safety, which is her object in preferring men-midwives, to be herself the occasion of temptation to those people? How can she answer that she will not be it? In that so formidable army of mercenaries, actually continuing to form itself under the banners of Fashion, and headed by Interest, can she answer that the insensible stoics of it, will fall to her share? Would a woman, I will not say, of strict principles of honor, but barely of not the most abandoned ones, submit herself in the manner she must to a man-midwife, on her employing him, if she would but satisfy herself, as she easily may, that his aid cannot be more effectual than that of a woman? But what! If it is most undoubtedly a less safe one?

But this is far from all to be objected on the head of modesty to this practice. The opportunities, if not of temptation, if not of seduction by it, at least of offensiveness to female reserve are such, as would make even a husband, the least susceptible of jealousy, so uneasy for the outrages to which the employing of a man-midwife in the course of his wife's pregnancy and delivery might expose her, as would make him think it no indifferent point for his judgment to settle whether such outrages might not better be spared her. It will not I presume be denied, that all female modesty is a flower, the delicacy of which cannot be too much guarded against any tendency to blast it, and that nothing can threaten more that effect, than such infringements of the unity of a husband's privilege in the sole uncommunicable possession of his wife's body, as are implied in the course of a man-midwife's attendance. An unity of privilege, which, when broke in one point; does not always stop at that, but may proceed to farther breach, where there is art on one side, and weakness on the other. Many women are doubtless proof against the slipperiness of such an overture: but all have not alike strength of mind.

But left I should be here taxed with forging of phantoms merely for the honor of combating them, I shall only entreat all parties concerned to consider the following so probable circumstance, and then let them decide as their own judgment will direct them: a circumstance taken (can any thing be fairer?) even from a man-midwife's own stating, as well as from the nature of things, of which none need be ignorant that will think at all about them.

It is then to be observed, that during a woman's pregnancy, and before the labor-pains come on, one of the principal points of midwifery is, what is called the art of *Touching*. Thence are derived the surest prognostics for preparation, and especially from the signs it affords of rectitude or obliquity of the Uterus. I have already offered reasons needless to repeat, why the men can never arrive at the excellence of skill in the women in this particular. But as to the importance of this faculty of *Touching*, hear what Dr. Smellie himself says.

P. 180. "The design of *touching* is to be informed, whether the woman is or is not with child; to know how far she is advance in her pregnancy; if she is in danger of a miscarriage; if the *os uteri* be dilated; and in time of labor to form a right judgment of the case, from the opening of the *os internum*, and the pressing down of the membranes with their waters, and lastly, to distinguish what part of the child is presented."

Again, p. 448. speaking of a *midwife*, he says, "she ought to be well skilled in the art of *touching* pregnant women, and know in what matter the womb stretches, together with the situation of all the abdominal VISCERA: she ought to be perfectly mistress of the ART of EXAMINATION in the time of labour".

Here you have from an unsuspected authority a certainly not over-rated importance of the expedience of preliminary TOUCHING. Now granting, only for argument's sake, what is assuredly false, that a man-practitioner can be equal (superior he would not in this point, at least, have the impudence to pretend himself) to a midwife; let a husband, let a wife, but reflect on the difference, every thing else being equal, there must be as to *modesty*, between the function of *touching* being performed by a man or by a woman. Let a husband, I say, for an instant figure to himself what a figure he must make, what a figure his wife must make, under such a ceremony performed by a lusty HE-MIDWIFE, exploring those arcana of the female fabric, and especially to so little purpose, with his natural disqualifications for so much as knowing what he is about. Will the husband be present? What must be the wife's confusion during so nauseous and so gross a scene? Will he *modestly* withdraw while his wife is so *served*? What must be his wife's danger from one of those rummagers, if she should be handsome enough to deserve his attention, or a compliment from him on such a visitation of her secret charms, the more flattering from *him*, not only as he must be supposed so good a judge from the frequency of his occasions of comparison, but as it must imply a superior corporal merit in the woman so visited, as could overcome that satiety which a fastidious plenty of patients might so naturally be imagined to create in a man-midwife? Will any one say, that these suppositions are over-strained, or out of Nature? I fancy, that if the secret histories of many families were ransacked, of the practice on which the men-midwives were in possession, it would not be always found, that those preliminary visitations were not turned to some account of interest or seduction. And yet an omission of that *touching* might be dangerous. How kind is it then in Nature, to have of herself so far consulted the good and tranquility of society, in palpably bestowing upon women a faculty, which she has as palpably refused to the men, in whom the exercise of it would for obvious reasons be big with so many inconveniences? Is there any breach of charity in the taking for granted the existence of such inconveniences, unless indeed, all of a sudden, in favor of this lucre-begotten sect, the men were ceased to be men, and the women women?

But allowing that nothing was to pass between a man-midwife and his patient, in this *act* of *touching*, beyond the necessity of the practice, or in a merely technical sense, that in short no such libertine impression should make itself be felt in the course of such *touches*, as should discompose the good *Doctor*'s DIGNITY, and endanger the patient's honor, by present or future attempts derived from such a strange privity; is it not to be feared, that a designing or interested person may take other advantages besides that of gratifying sensuality? May not a woman, the more attached she is to her modesty, the greater sacrifice she has made of it, in her innocence of intention, only imagine herself but the more subjected to a man, to whom she has submitted in the manner she must do to a man-midwife, and let him take an ascendant over her and her family, of which a midwife would not so much as dream, from her office being so much in course, and too little extraordinary for her to have any extraordinary pretentions or designs? On the contrary, a man-midwife need scarce set any bounds to his. In any differences in a family, especially between man and wife, must not a man-practitioner, from such a familiarity with the wife's person, have such a footing in the confidence of the wife, as may enable him to dispose of her will almost in any thing? He may be her apothecary, physician, surgeon, privy-councellor, what not? What can a woman refuse a man, to whom she is so deluded as to think she owes her own life, or that of a darling child, all his merit, in which I have before explained? What can a woman in short refuse a man, to whom nothing of that has been refused, in which consist all the preliminaries of granting every thing? She may indeed refuse him the sacrifice of her virtue, if he should think it worth

106

designing upon, but how few things else could she refuse him? Once more the greater value she put on the sacrifice of so much of her modesty, the less would she be able to deny him any thing else, as any thing else must comparatively appear so inconsiderable.

But hitherto I have spoke only of those outrages and dangers to modesty from the preparatory attendance of the man-midwife as occasion may require, during the pregnancy. But as to his officiating in the crisis of the labor-pains and delivery, there are two very essential points of consideration.

The first. The modesty of the women, unaccustomed to the approaches of other men than a husband, must be in great sufferance in the moments of their labor-pains. All Nature agonizes in them. They are at once weakened in the flesh and in the spirit. The bare presence of a man to officiate at such a time, may excite in them a revolution capable of stopping the labor-pains caused by the expulsive efforts of delivery, which thus becomes dangerously retarded, and may so overpower them, as to put them in the greatest peril of their lives. This is what has often happened. You may see frequent examples of this revolt of Nature against the ministry of men-midwives in Dr. La Motte himself, a man-midwife. If Nature then suffers so much in women at the juncture, when a person, nay even of the same sex, offers her aid, in certain indispensable occasions, to which humanity is subjected; how greatly must the presence of a man increase their constraint and embarrassment, and rob them still more of that so necessary freedom in the animal functions! But how greatly ought the women to thank that their instinctive repugnance of Nature to such a prostitution of their persons, if they consider those tortures, which, by the listening to that same repugnance, may at once be saved to their modesty, and to their personal feeling. Let them paint themselves the following posture prescribed by a man-midwife. "*The patient must be commodiously placed, that is to say, on the bed-side, her thighs raised and expanded, her feet drawn up to her posteriors, and kept steady in that posture by some trustly helpers.*"[25] Levret, p. 161. *On the use of the new crooked forceps.* Here it may be said; "why there is nothing in this attitude, however shockingly indecent, but what may be sanctified by the extremities of necessity". Very well. But what must a

---

[25] "Il faut d'abord placer convenablement la malade, c'est-a-dire, sur le bord de son lit; les cuisses elevees et ecartées, les pieds rapprochés des fesses, et maintenus en cette situation par des aides dont on soit sur." *Levret*, UTILITE DU NOUVEAU FORCEPS COUREE, p. 161.

husband, what must a wife think at her being *spread out* in this manner, under the hands and eyes of a man-practitioner, with his helpers, perhaps his trusty apprentices, only for the experiment of a *forceps* of a new invention, the merit of which too is a so contested an one, that Levret himself is forced to own that, "that same FORCEPS *"would be*[26] *an instrument of pure* SPECULATION, *and not of* PRACTICE, IF (N.B. that IF) *a certain general precept should be true*," which, by the by, is most certainly so! So that, in this case, for example, you see how a woman may be treated, only to ascertain the merit of some new-fangled gimcrack of an instrument. But to how many occasions of as little, or even less necessity than this, for putting a woman into postures of this sort, might not wantonness, interest, or other motives give birth? Or can pretexts for such insults to modesty be wanting to designingness?

The second consideration is this. Those moments of weakness of spirit, and infirmity to which the labor-pains subject the women may, in some of naturally the weakest of them be, liable to leave impressions in favor of a man-midwife, the less suspected of harm, and consequently the more dangerous for their being suggested by that gratitude for his imaginary[27] contribution to their deliverance, which is itself a virtue, though the object of it is so miserably mistaken by them. Let any one image to himself what must often happen in Nature, a woman sinking under her pains, her mind all softened and overpowered with her present feelings, and looking up for *relief* to the *man*, employed, as she imagines, to procure it her, though the real fact oftenest is,

---

[26] "Si on s'arrêtoit au precepte general, le *forceps* seroit un instrument de pure speculation et non de pratique." Lev. p. 161.

[27] The term *imaginary* is here far from an unjust one, and why should not the honor of a deliverance, effectuated by Nature, be as well given to a being of flesh and blood as to a stone? The virtue of the *ætites*, or Eagle-stone, has currently passed for abridging the pains of labor, and accelerating purturition. A French consul in Egypt, ordered one of those stones to be tied to his wife's thigh, who was in a lingering labor. The stone in this case, more innocent than probably a man-midwife would have been, who would have used means to hurry the birth, or perhaps have gone to work with his *forceps* at least, suffered Nature quietly to go her own pace. What was the consequence? The lady was soon after happily delivered, which there is no doubt but she would equally have been if a brick-bat had been tied to her thigh. But Nature lost the thanks so justly due to her: the stone ran away with all her merit; and this case was added to the catalogue of the miraculous operations of the stone. In how many cases might it be said, that the stone here represents the man-midwife, if to the stone it was not so much more innocent and less dangerous to have a recourse?

that he will not have enough prevented her pain, or perhaps greatly occasioned its increase. Of this however she knowing nothing, sees him in the amiable light of her deliverer from her actual and intolerable state of pain. In the mean time, those aukward uncouth endeavours of his to relieve and deliver her, even though they should aggravate her torture, pass upon her for master-pieces of art or skill. "Who would be without a man-midwife?" At length, Nature sometimes, even in spite of all his omissions, or bungled operation, proceeds in her favorite task of delivery, that is to say, if he has not hurried or made tragic work of it, with his mis-practice of his instruments. The patient then is rid of her burthen, and what are then her feelings? Those of exquisite delight, from the comparison with what she was induring but the instant before. It is a transport of joy, not unmingled with gratitude, to the person to whom she fancies herself in any measure obliged for it. The ugliest wretch on earth, so he could but be imagined the cause of such a delivery, would, in those instants, assume in her eyes the form of Loveliness itself. Even with the greatest innocence of heart she could hug, she could kiss him in the ebullitions of her joy and gratitude. Let no one imagine these expressions are over-strained. Such a rapture of felicity, in the sudden case of being taken as it were down from a rack, is not of a Nature to know any bounds of moderation, nor can be conceived but by those who have felt it. Her gratitude would even extend do inanimate things, much more to the dear Doctor, to whom she conceives she owes so much. She eyes him with all the intense eagerness of a gratitude so fond, that its transiency into a passion of another nature would not appear such a prodigy, to those who consider how apt passions of tenderness are to confound motives and run into one another. The melting-softness of those moments of infirmity and weakness of spirit, affords a susceptibility of impressions, which may not afterwards be so soon worn out, and of which the usual affection from the difference of sexes, in the parties, may sooner or later come in for its share. Dr. Smellie has, as I have before observed, implicity allowed the possibility of a temptation to men, and shall I not follow his laudable example of candor, and confess that there may also be weak women?

It is indeed true that in cases of extremities, such as most certainly are not the frequentest ones, any thought of immodesty may be intirely out of the question. The sad and suffering state of a woman agonizing with pain, at the gates one may say of death, leaves little room for licentious temptations. But, once more, those cases are much the rarest: and even in those, the greater the danger will have been, the greater must the gratitude afterwards be for the imaginary service, that will be supposed to have accomplished the deliverance. Let a midwife have really rendered that service, the gratitude will scarce be so quick, so lively or so lasting, only because she is not a man.

If it shall be here objected, that the men-midwives ought to be above all suspicion or scandal of this sort; I shall only say, that at least it is their interest to appear so. But they themselves will not pretend to an exemption from temptation, nor can answer for themselves that such a temptation may not come into existence, as that all their virtue, fortified by the divine precept before quoted from Dr. Smellie, may not defend them from yielding to it. They are not, or at least ought not to be men in years for obvious reasons as to that manual practice of theirs which at the best is so indifferent. Let any one then consider the consequence of this worse than unnecessarily putting young women, in such manner, into the hands of men in the vigor of their age. Let any impartial person but reflect what barriers are thrown down, what a door is opened to licentiousness, by the admission of this so perfectly needless innovation. Think of an army, if but of barely Dr. Smellie's nine-hundred pupils, constantly recruiting with the pupils of those pupils, let loose against the female sex, and of what an havock they make of both its safety and modesty, to say nothing of the detriment to population, in the destruction of infants, and I presume, it will not appear intirely in me a suggestion of private interest to wish things, in this point, restored to the old course of practice of this art of midwifery by women. A course which Nature has so self-evidently established, in her tender regard to the female sex, and to its darling offspring, and in which she has not less consulted one of her primary ends, the Good of Society, in the greater security of the conjugal union and property, which ought to be so sacred, and especially so, for the honor of the human understanding, from the invasion of an upstart profession, sordidly mean in its motives, infamously false in its pretences, shamefully ridiculous in its practice, and yet dreadfully serious in all its consequences.

CONCLUSION OF THE FIRST PART.

In the foregoing part of this work I have contented myself with asserting, in general, the perfect inutility of those instruments, of which the male-practitioners themselves confess the danger, and use them not a bit the less for that confession. It is then for the following and second part, that I have reserved the entering into a more particular discussion of them. Therein will appear, upon how false and slender a foundation the gentlemen-midwives have insinuated themselves into a business so little made for them. The truth is, that the pernicious quackery of those same instruments has been artfully made the pretext, and become the sanction of an innovation set on foot by Interest, adopted by Credulity, and at length fostered by Fashion. The employing of midwives was undoubtedly not long since, in this country, the General Rule. The calling in of men-practitioners, upon very extraordinary occasions, was an Exception, and a very rare one, to that General Rule. But by a fatal inversion of the natural order of things, the Exception is recently crept into the place of the General Rule. The point is to consider, whether this palpable violence to Nature is of that benefit to society which it is pretended to be.

I have already examined some of the arguments in favor of the men-practitioners. But the principal one, deduced from the incapacity, or rather aversion of the midwives, upon just grounds, from using instruments, merits an ampler scrutiny. In proof of my candor in it, I shall take most of my remarks on those instruments from what the men-practitioners themselves say, and confess of them. This, I presume, cannot be deemed unfair.

Upon the whole, those parties whom the decision may concern, will please to decide on which side the force of Reason and Truth shall appear the greatest; and so deciding, it is, in fact, in their own favor, and in one of their most capital concerns, that they will decide.

They will decide, in short, whether, upon the whole, the plea of the men-practitioners, sounded upon the ignorance of a few midwives which, bad as it is, is more than balanced by their incompetency in the manual function, and to which a remedy might easily be found, is a valid one for driving out of the practice of midwifery a sex, to which the faculty of it is self-evidently the genuine gift of Nature herself, only to make way for a set of interested male-practitioners, whose so boasted art is oftenest signalized by the most barbarous

111

and horrid outrages upon Nature, with this aggravation, that they are needlessly committed under the specious and plausible pretext of flying to her assistance.

THE END OF THE FIRST PART.

PART THE SECOND.

Containing various observations on the labor and delivery of lying-in women, including a discussion of the pretended necessity for the employing instruments.

INTRODUCTION.

NOTWITHSTANDING the numerous productions of writers on the art of succoring women in labor, all that has hitherto appeared on that subject, still leaves the mind unsatisfied; not that it is so unjust as to expect perfection in any human art, but from its feeling that, in this particular one, too much is given to theory, and too little to the practical part, or manual function.

While the causes of difficult labors are far from solidly or sufficiently explained, and rather obscured by a cloud of scientific jargon, than practically illustrated, they give us no tolerably sure method for preventing or remedying those difficulties. On the contrary, the whole boasted improvement of the art is reduced, to a pernicious recourse to instruments, which cut at once the knot they cannot unty.

It is then no wonder that there should still, in all the books and observations hitherto given on this matter, exist a void lamentably unfilled; and as this void evidently consist less in the theory than the practice, the superior qualifications, and natural endowments of the women for the manual operation, point out the fitness of the greater dependence on them for the filling up what, humanly speaking, can be filled up of that void.

Let the physicians, the surgeons instruct the midwives in so much of anatomy as is necessary to their function; let them afford them, either in writing or verbally, their guidance and direction in the consequences or occasionally in the preliminaries of management of the lying-in; all this is right, salutary, and in due course: but that men should pretend to the manual operation in these cases, it certainly neither is nor can be their business. Nor is this negation of propriety a reproach to them. Will any man think it an

113

indignity to be told, he cannot clear-starch, hem a ruffle, or make a bed as handily as a woman? The exceptions are the shame; and in this department of art it would be truer to say, that there are no exceptions than that there are only a few.

But can we wonder at the insufficiency of the lights thrown into the art of midwifery by that of writers who have treated of it, when so few of them having had any other view than advertising themselves, and being incapable of saying any thing to the purpose, of the art of delivering the women, have filled up their books with insignificant digressions, or things intirely foreign from the point?

In some you see all distempers of women collateral to their pregnancy, which is certainly a very necessary and an infinitely extensive subject, while on the practical article of the deliverance they give you nothing but what is barren, jejune, or even false. Others, by way of filling up, run digressively into a discussion of the methods of treating infants. Others again have written only to recommend some pretended secrets, as powders, preparations, &c. Some have swelled their volumes with the more or less commodious structure of a couch, or the mechanism of a close-stool, or the make of different sorts of syringes for anodine injections. In others you meet with remedies for the deformities of the human body, for the contractions or stiffnesses of the muscles of the shoulders, arms, hands, legs, feet, thighs, haunches, &c. to straiten the crooked, and even, in a treatise on midwifery, to extirpate a polypus from the nose. Others, with all the parade of justly exclaiming against nostrum-mongers, the plausible writing against which serves at once to fill up, and give them an air of superiority to such trumpery, substitute however nothing better of their own than the recommendation of some instrument, which they give you for a master-piece of invention; and to establish which, they cry down every instrument of other practitioners, though not one jot inferior to it in any thing, but the not being the newest. Thus, after having perused such a multiplicity of authors, it is incredible to say how little true, or practically useful knowledge is to be picked out of the whole mass of them. You find almost every thing in them but what you are looking for.

In the mean time, the superficial examiner of things, who sees such a number of volumes, furnished by these pretenders to the art of midwifery, cannot conceive they contain matter so little essential as they do. The scientific

114

air diffused over them, not a little embellished with pretty prints of machines, as of a windowed forceps, a stool, or of a gravid uterus, all these contribute to throw the dust or erudition into the eyes of those, who do not penetrate beyond the surface of things. And thus the aids and appendages of the art, or what is yet worse, even the abuses of it, pass for the art itself, the main of which, as it undoubtedly consists in the expertness or dexterity of the manual practice, can be so little and so imperfectly conveyed by description. I am however far from denying the benefit which may result to midwives, from consulting all that has been written on this subject. I am far from encouraging ignorance in the women of this profession. Their skill in the manual function cannot but be improved by the addition of a sound and competent theory. But it should always be remembered, that the very basis or capital point of the art is the manual dexterity; and in that point, the most learned of the men must yield to the most ignorant of the women. A point which the mens surpassing the women in every thing else can never compensate: no not with all those dreadful "artificial hands", of which they boast so much their invention, in the room of the infinitely perferably *natural* ones, of which the use, in this office, becomes the men as little, as their hands seem formed for it; and I might add, their heads, if they themselves can possibly think otherwise. In such an opinion the ignorance is theirs.

As to the treatise herein offered on the art of midwifery, as the object of it is principally to attack particular abuses and dangerous innovations in it, it will not be expected that the same should furnish a complete general course of practice. But this I dare aver that if I should be induced to attempt such a work, it will not be the worse for my consulting more the experience I have of Nature in her operations in this one of her so capital concerns, than the authorities of men, who seem or pretend to know so little of her, as to think of assisting her with instruments, formed only for her destruction, or at least for doing her more damage by their violence, than any reason to hope good from them can justify.

Here I shall not offer any digressions on physic, anatomy, chemistry, or pharmacy; I shall confine myself entirely to the points of my business of the manual operation. Let the physician prescribe, the surgeon bleed, the chymist contribute medicines, the apothecary make them up; with none of these professions do I presume to interfere. But as to the man-midwife, who not only so often presumes in some measure to represent them all, but to join to them the exercise of an art so unnatural to his sex, I should think myself wanting to my duty in my profession, if I did not point out the mischief I apprehended to result from especially that method of practice, on which he grounds the pretence of necessity for his practising it at all; and this chiefly forms the object of this second part, in supplement to my first.

OF DELIVERIES.

We understand, by deliveries, in general, the issue of the fœtus out of the mother's womb.

These are distinguished into two kinds, the one natural, the other preternatural.

The natural one, is that in which the fœtus comes out in the most ordinary way, when it presents the head foremost.

It is deemed preternatural, when the fœtus presents in the passage any other part than the head.

These two kinds are again subdivided into two distinctions of labor, of easy or difficult, because both the natural and preternatural mode of delivery may be easy or difficult.

The delivery is termed easy when the fœtus comes out readily, and without the aid of art.

It is termed difficult, when the labor of it is hard, and the fœtus does not make its way out but with pain, and with the help and assistant industry of the midwife.

In the cases of a natural and easy delivery, there is little or no actual occasion for the presence of the midwife, beyond that of receiving the fœtus, tying the navel-string, giving the child to be kept warm, and then delivering the mother of the after-birth. The spirits of patient are then to be recomposed, her agitation calmed, a warm and soft linnen cloth applied to the stomach; a warm shift and bed-gown put on her; a linnen cloth to be laid on four-fold over the belly; a double-napkin round her, and she to be placed in a bed well warmed. Such is the summary of the process to be observed in those common cases.

In the deliveries, on a preternatural labor, when they are easy, the same method takes place: there being no difference, but that in one the child will have been received by the head, in the other by the feet.

These kinds of labors are so easy, that there is no need of demonstrating their being to be terminated without the aid of instruments. When the fœtus presents itself promisingly, Nature is best left to her own action, and nothing should be precipitated in the manual function, unless some unexpected accident should intervene, and require interposition, such as a great flooding, or other exigency.

As to the preternatural delivery, the better practice is not to delay the extraction of the fœtus, after the discharge of the waters; nor stay till her strength shall have been exhausted. On the presenting of a fair hold, and a sufficient overture, no difficulty should be made of extracting.

All that is to be observed then, is not to prematurate this extraction: not to proceed, in short, like those unskilful, or inconsiderate practitioners, who are no sooner entered the patient's room, but they want to have their operation dispatched out of hand. Nothing can be more important to the well-doing of the patient, than for no violence to be used to Nature, who loves to go her own full time, without disturbance or molestation. In this point then great caution and circumspection are requisite.

It should also be observed, that it is wrong for the midwife to leave a woman newly lain-in, however happily delivered. It is necessary to stay by her for some hours afterwards, till she is in such a state of tranquility and ease, as may leave nothing to fear of those after-disasters which too often happen.

Some celebrated practitioners and authors upon midwifery have been surprized to see women, after their going their time without mis-adventure, and after having been readily and happily brought to bed die suddenly. There are too many of both the female and the men-midwives who have no notion of this misfortune till it is too late to prevent it. The cause of this melancholic accident is unknown to many practitioners of the art. Some have confessed their ignorance of it: others have erroneously, others deficiently accounted for it. But all are surprized when the patient is the victim of it: especially as it follows, in some cases that afford the best grounded hopes.

Messieurs Mauriceau and De la Motte give us examples of these unexpected deaths. The first, in his 230th observation, says,

"I delivered a woman of a very corpulent habit, aged about thirty-five years, of her first child, which was a lusty girl, alive, and that came naturally. This woman had been near two days in labor, with small slow pains or throws, after which the waters having burst forth with a strong throw, she had subsequently favorable ones, which made her bring forth as happily as one could wish. I immediately delivered her: but to my great surprize, scarce had she been a quarter of an hour after delivery, that she of a sudden fell into violent faintings, with an oppression at the breast, and a great agitation of the whole body, which was instantly followed by a convulsion, caused by a loss of blood, of which she died a quarter of an hour afterwards.

This (adds Mr. Mauriceau) was one of those kind of fatalities which no human prudence can elude or parry."

La Motte had the same case happened under his hands; which I need not repeat here, being inserted in the first part of this work, where, p. 131, I ventured to promise an essay of mine, to give a less unsatisfactory reason of such deaths, than what is to be found even in those two celebrated authors whom our contemporaries consider as their masters in the art of midwifery. These impute those unforeseen deaths to occult and inevitable *causes*. I own, I do not intirely think them either occult or inevitable. I doubtless may be mistaken, but of this I am sure, I shall advance nothing but what is authenticated to me by my own observation and experience.

An over-repletion of blood; and a defect in the contraction of the uterus, of which all the vessel being open are too slow in recovering their occlusion, are generally speaking, the causes of these diseases. I could support this opinion by some chirurgical axioms, but I presume it will be thought more satisfactory proved by the success of the method of practice, which I would recommend to prevent or cure those dangerous or rather fatal causes.

As to know that a woman may thus perish unexpectedly a quarter of an hour after delivery, is enough to require the being on one's guard for using a salutary prevention; I would advise attention, especially to her constitution.

Whenever therefore a pregnant woman is observed to be remarkably corpulent, and full of blood, with a good constitution, she should be advised to lose some blood, once or twice during her pregnancy, by way of precaution. This is of great service to rarefy the blood, and obviate those excessive hemorrhages, which are to be dreaded on their lying-in. Then nothing is to be precipitated during their labors, that Nature may have full time to predispose the uterus to enter into contraction by due degrees, that is to say, neither too quick, not too slow. But if, notwithstanding these precautions, there should, after delivery, supervene any considerable loss of blood, followed with faintings or oppressions, the patient must be stirred, excited to cough and sneeze contributively to the evacuation of the blood, which otherwise is apt to clot in the uterus, and would suffocate her if not expelled.

If by this mean the evacuation does not naturally take place, which may be perceived by the faintings of the patient, the midwife must, without losing time, put her hand into the bowel, and extract all the clots of blood she will not fail of finding there, and of which the presence, as being extraneous matter, necessarily oppose the contraction of this organ, and quickly suffocates the woman, if she is not timely relieved.

These hemorrhages are but too frequent, especially with those women who neglect the precautionary bleeding; and such sudden death too commonly the consequence of neglecting, or of not knowing that the most salutary practice, in these cases, is to well evacuate the uterus by the operation of the hand, where Nature appears in the least tardy or deficient.

The long experience I have of this manual help, which has never failed of success with me, warrants my averring, that there is little or no danger, in these cases, to women, provided the midwife employs herself dexterously to clear them while time serves. Their relief is instantaneous. They come to themselves presently: they are restored to a freedom of respiration: nor will they have so much as been sensible of this operation of the hand, which will nevertheless have saved their lives.

There have been men-midwives, that pass even for learned, but who from their ignorance of this so simple and easy method of relief, have been in the disagreeable circumstance of seeing many women perish under their hands, though they had to all appearance been very happily delivered.

With respect to pregnant women, there is again another point of great consequence to ascertain. Great care must be taken not to mistake the signs of delivery. This is a very essential matter. Nothing scarce can be more dangerous, than to excite a woman to the last labor-pains, which will not fail of exhausting that strength of her's, in vain, which had so much better be reserved for the support of her in the time she will really need it. So that a

119

midwife ought to make it her business clearly to distinguish the spurious pains from the true ones. Where a woman near her time feels pains in the belly, the loins, or even the sexual parts; they are not always to be taken for the true labor-pains. In this point, the *touching* will be a great guidance.

If the fœtus is still high in the uterus, and the situation of it does not indicate a readiness for extrusion; if the waters are not sufficiently prepared, or their pressure down not in due forwardness, the pains must be assuaged by some calming anodine remedies: the patient must be left to her rest, till things declare themselves more openly; and then, as she will not have been fruitlessly fatigued and tormented, the labor may proceed happily.

There have been men-practitioners so very unskilful, or at a loss for delivering women by the operation of their *hands*, that they tortured their *heads* to discover *medicines* to save themselves the tediousness of Nature's taking her own time, as if she was to do her work the better for their hurrying her. Towards the achievement of this end, they brought into play certain drugs, to which they gave the appellation of hysteric, and placed or pretended to place great confidence in them.

Even some of our modern practitioners prove, at least, by their practice, that they have faith in the virtue of such drugs, since they continue to use them. They are still suffered to make a figure in many of the Pharmacopœas, though no sure experience hitherto has verified their efficacy. On the contrary, a thousand and a thousand examples might be quoted in demonstration of their insufficiency and danger. I shall content myself with producing here the testimony of Mr. De la Motte, in the second book of his observations, and he is not the only man-midwife that does such medicines the justice of disapproving them.

OBSERVATION 174.

"A celebrated man-midwife of this town (says Mr. de la Motte) pretended to have a marvellous powder to provoke labor-pains, and accelerate parturition. This powder was composed of galbanum, myrrh, savin, rue, and other drugs, of which he made the patient take a dose, to hasten a delivery, when the labor was lingering, from half a drachm to a drachm, and after the effect of this medicine, which ended commonly in leaving the patient in a worse condition than before the taking it, he substituted the use of the crotchet, which was indeed an infallible method of putting a speedy end to the labor; and of which he as well as his fellow-practitioners made such a murderous use, the aid of the hand well conducted being unknown to them.

"The same operator (says Mr. de la Motte) was sent for to assist a lady who had continued in labour for three days, to whom he proposed a dose of his powders, to which she readily consented in the hopes of a speedy delivery. Unluckily, not most certainly for the lady, but for the honor of the powders, the operator, not having had the providence of having them about him, was forced to go home for them. The lady, in the mean while, was brought very happily to bed, just as he was re-entering the room with his dose for her. What a pity this was! What would not have been the boast of the virtue of those pretious powders, if the delivery had waited for them but half a quarter of an hour, though they would not have had the least share in it, since it would have been purely the work of Nature and Time.

"This celebrated man-midwife was called to two other women of my acquaintance, of whom the labor somewhat resembled that of this lady, but of which the consequences were very different: he had made them take his powders to no manner of purpose, when seeing that a day had passed without their producing the expected effect, he had recourse to his *crotchet*, with which he quickly *dispatched* both the deliveries."

OBSERVATION 174, OF THE SAME MR. DE LA MOTTE.

"A gentleman who lived upon his fortune, without professing surgery, though he had served his time to it, and had even formerly exercised it, not only in France, but in Italy, and in other foreign countries, told me, in conversation, that he had an infallible remedy to make a woman bring forth instantaneously, however lingering and difficult her labor might naturally be. Of this, he said, he had made undoubted experiments, and that he had obtained this secret from an Italian, under oath of not disclosing it to any one. He was more than a little surprized at finding me without curiosity to learn from him this pretended secret, which he imagined must concern me so much, as one who made open profession of the obstetrical art; and still greater was his surprize at seeing me change the subject, without any sign of attention to what he had been saying on this head."

"In process of time, he married, and his wife being pregnant was got into the time of her labor-pains towards delivery. It became now expedient for him to declare this famous secret to me, which was no other than half a drachm of borax in a glass of any innocent liquid agreeable to the palate of the patient. But as this dose happened to be administered by one who had no sort of faith in it, it had no effect: his wife lay four days and four nights in labor; the child died the moment after it was born, and the mother narrowly escaped following it.

OBSERVATION 176, (OF M. DE LA MOTTE)

"As I was at Caën, a town of Normandy, attending the lying-in of a lady there, an old stander of a practitioner of that place, and a man of good abilities, told me, that he had been lately sent for to a woman who had continued several days in labor, with slow and moderate pains. As he found the fœtus well situated, he made the patient take an infusion of three drachms of sena in the juice of a seville orange, in order to quicken the throws and advance the delivery, which indeed came on ten or twelve hours afterwards, but the woman died, one may say, immediately after it.

"To this account (continues M. De la Motte) I opposed, for answer, that being at Bayeux, on the like occasion, an old practitioner in surgery of that place, in conjunction with whom I had been called to visit a patient, told me, in conversation, that he understood midwifery very well, that he had even, not long before terminated a delivery given over by another surgeon; that the child, one arm of which hung out, was dead, before he put his hand to it, and that the mother, though well delivered, died soon after."

These examples may suffice to prove, that the notion of giving histeric medicines, for which the inventors did not forget to make themselves be well paid, existed in M. De la Motte's time, who is not but a modern author: nor are they even to this hour absolutely exploded, tho' some of the men-midwives themselves have joined Mr. de la Motte's cry against them. It gives however those men-practitioners, who exclaim against a quackery in others, by which themselves get nothing, a good sort of an air: it serves even to render that more pernicious quackery of their instruments the less obnoxious to suspicion. Nothing is easier to give up than that by which nothing is got. If the instruments were not a plea for the very essence of such a thing as a man-midwife, they too would be given up. However, it will hardly be denied, that those same pompous histeric medicines were the invention of *learned* men-practitioners, and not of those poor ignorant midwives, who, with respect to women in labor, are of opinion, that there can nothing be more effectual for their well-doing, than in the first place giving Nature fair-play, and, when requisite, to assist her with the management of *natural* hands skilfully conducted: always observing neither to lapse nor precipitate the critical time of such assistance. In the mean time, let a humane reader but reflect how many mothers and children must have been, and perhaps still continue to be the victims of a reliance in such medicines, and he will allow, that such errors of practice, tho' not capital in the intention, are too often deplorably so in the effect. Is it not true to say, considering the havock of the human species, so presumably made by quackery and empiricism in general, that the lives of the subject are less sacred than their property? Surely they are less guarded, either by the laws, or by common sense.

As to a fœtus that presents an arm, or any other part than the head or feet, there is rarely any thing to do but to slide the hand all along that arm, or other part it may present, to find out the feet, and terminate the delivery; without its being necessary to attempt the reduction of any part or member.

Most of the writers on midwifery often start difficulties where there are really none. They often give us emphatical accounts of a head too large, and a passage too narrow, in which they state them as difficulties that are invincible, when the case is far from being so. When the fœtus presents fair, and is in a good posture, our method of practice is, to advise the patient to remain as quiet a-bed as possible, avoiding every thing that may tend to fatigue her body, or hurry her spirits, to reserve in short her strength as much as possible. With time and patience the head of the fœtus scarcely ever fails of moulding itself to the passage, through a particular providence of Nature, which has so ordered it, that the parietal bones of the head of the fœtus, so flexile as to ride over one another, form a kind of oval figure, which facilitates the issue, and dispose it for making way for itself, through the extrusive pressure of the labor-throws. Mean while nothing should be done to irritate the pains; the membranes should not be unnecessarily or untimely burst, which loses the benefit of the waters. You can hardly, in this case, rely too much on the benevolent efforts of Nature: she is constantly at work for the patient's delivery. Interruptions sometimes only serve to mar or retard a favorable crisis: but all abrupt force or violence is carefully to be avoided. As to bad postures of children, I shall treat of them in the sequel, and of the means to remedy them.

OF DIFFICULT AND SEVERE CASES.

If an easy delivery requires nothing of extraordinary assistance; it is not so with a difficult one. All the knowledge, experience, dexterity, strength, prudence, tenderness, charity, and presence of mind, of which a woman is capable, are requisite to accomplish certain laborious deliveries.

It has been, in all times, very well known, that the most natural situation for the fœtus coming into the world, is that, in which the head presents first, it being that which commonly makes way for the rest of the body. Yet this delivery may become difficult, in proportion to the obstacles incident to it: obstacles not always surmountable, without great skill and industry employed in aid of Nature.

On the other hand, when it is felt that the fœtus presents any other part than the head, this position, called preternatural, oftenest occasions the delivery to be more laborious and hard to accomplish, in proportion to the more or less trouble there may be to scarch and come rightly at the feet.

Many English and French authors have given us a long enumeration of the causes which may make deliveries difficult and laborious. The curious may have recourse to them; as for me, who have not proposed to myself here a treatise compleat on all points, I shall content myself with setting forth only what tends to fullfil my proposed aim, that is to say, to take notice of those principal points, which first moved insufficient midwives to call in surgery to their assistance, to remedy their blunders, to retrieve their mischief, or to repair their omissions. I shall consider the kinds of exigencies, which the men-operators seized for a pretext of employing their iron and steel-instruments, the use of the natural hand, being yet more unknown to them than to the meanest midwife, and by this means, for the cure of confessedly a great evil, obtruded an infinitely greater one, and more extensive, in every sense, and in every point of light, that of men taking the practical part of midwifery into their own hands, or rather into their artificial ones of iron and steel, from which they derive all the authority of their introduction in the character of men-midwives.

124

The labors then which are generally speaking looked on the most nice, and arduous, may be comprized under the following heads.

1st. The obliquity of the uterus or womb.

2dly. The extraction of the head of the fœtus severed from the body, and which shall have remained in the uterus.

3dly. That labor in which the head of the fœtus remains hitched in the passage, the body being intirely come out of the uterus.

4thly. When the head of the fœtus presents itself foremost, but sticks in the passage.

To these I shall add the case of the pendulous belly, which is not without its difficulty.

Of all these classes of labors I shall treat separately. But before I proceed on them, I presume, that it may not be improper preliminarily to corroborate what I have said of the intrusion of the men into the practice of a profession, of the essential part of which they were so ignorant and disqualified for it, by the testimony which one of the best men-midwives in Europe has not refused to the truth.

This is M. de la Motte, one of the ablest and most intelligent modern writers on the subject of midwifery, of which his works form an incontestable proof. The ingenuity and candor with which he has written, must render him less suspected than any other. This is no midwife. He is a man, and esteemed an able practitioner, who learned the principles of the art of Madam la Marche, head-midwife of the Hôtel Dieu at Paris. He made his advantage of the works of his predecessors Mauriceau, Peu, and of all the best authors on this subject. All that was worth it in them he has transfused into his own writings; and that in a very clear manner. He collected whatever the best phisicians had usefully said on the diseases of mother and child: in short, he has added many good observations and reflexions of his own, in the journals of his manual practice: the reading of his works, with some precaution however, cannot but be useful to the students of the art.

I do this writer this justice, with the more readiness and pleasure, for, that though he himself exercised the profession of man-midwife, and consequently in favor of his own practice, and of the pupils he was bringing up, was not without the injustice of adopting the prejudices of his contemporaries too indiscriminately against the midwives; he does not suppress any truth relative to the art itself. But even, as to the midwives, the truth escapes him without any design on his side of its coming out. But such is the force of truth. And thus it appears. M. De la Motte wrote in a little sorry country-town at a great distance from the capital, being at the very extremity of the kingdom of France, on a sea-coast, where there were no other midwives than poor country-women, without knowledge, without skill, or any other qualification, than a little of the habit of attending women in labor. Yet with all these deficiencies it will appear, that the men-practitioners were far more to be dreaded than those poor ignorant creatures, who had scarce any thing but Nature for their guide.

I shall here give the substance of what he says in his preface, followed by some examples of the unskilfulness, or rather of the most profound ignorance of the most able men-midwives of his time, for forty leagues round his place of residence in the country.

"It is (says M. De la Motte) astonishing, that the obstetrical art should, until the beginning of the preceding age, have been left either to ignorant women, or to surgeons, who had not (any more than too many to this day) any other resource in difficult labors, than some instrument guided by undextrous hands, always sure of killing the child, and endangering the mother. Do not these poor innocents deserve compassion for being exposed to operations of surgery, which one would rationally think they could not need, till providence should have at least given them leave to come into the world?"

Here be it observed, that by the word "ignorant," M. De la Motte should not intend the application of it to the midwives of the Hôtel Dieu at Paris, since, by his own confession, it is the best school of midwifery in Europe. Nor certainly is he in the wrong. Be it in honor of truth allowed me to say, that I know of those women who have served their apprenticeship in this hospital, who would think they made a wretched bargain, if they exchanged the manner of operating they learned there, for all the Latin, Greek, Arabic, or the iron and steel instruments of the best man-practitioner in Europe; even though his excellence in the manual function should be thrown into the scale for make-weight. The most constant success justifies their practice. In whatever situation the fœtus has presented, I have seen them, without having recourse to a man-midwife, and consequently to instruments, procure a happy delivery in very difficult labors. I have myself seen one deliver a child that had been dead in the mother's womb for near six weeks, without dismembering it; and though it was half-putrified, and the head so rotten-tender as to have no solid consistence, I dare advance this, without fear of being falsified, since I can name the mother, now alive in London, the witnesses, the place and year.

Such real midwives as I am here discribing, for I do not mean the spurious nominal ones, only fit to *create* work for the instrumentarians, or whose cue of interest is to do so, have no reason to apprehend, that in the numbers they have lain, there can be any found, that can complain of having suffered, or of suffering any the least damage or inconvenience, after their lying-in, that might be imputed to ignorance or mis-practice.

On the contrary, I dare aver, that such, genuine midwives have cured many women who had received notable injury, before they came under their hands, in their having passed through those of the men-practitioners. Nothing being more agreeable to Nature, to Reason, to Experience, than that the method of practice of a skilful midwife is not only the most easy and gentle, the least painful, but assuredly the most safe both for mother and child. This is what the most severe examination will to those, who give themselves the trouble of making it, establish, in contempt of that fashion, by which so pernicious an error, as that of preferring men-practitioners, has acquired more credit and influence than so salutary and demonstrable a truth, as that for which I am contending. In the mean time, let us hear what M. De la Motte himself, a man-midwife, says of those brethren of his, of whom heaven grant there may not exist to this day too many resemblers!

"To the shame (says M. de la Motte) of the profession they exercise, they have no guide but their avarice, while the grossest ignorance of the art of midwifery itself is their lot. Such are much to be dreaded by women in difficult labor; for (adds he) they having no help to offer them but that of their instruments, they employ them indifferently in all the situations in which the foetus presents. Nay, even the hands of some who will use their hands, are not less dangerous when misconducted. The ignorant therefore should never meddle with lyings-in. It would save them from the reproach they may incur of murder, in undertaking what they cannot execute, and what surpasses their skill. They would not furnish *scenes* that make one *shudder* with *horror*.

"I speak here of so many poor women, whose strength shall have been exhausted by a great loss of blood, caused by the violences which an ignorant man-midwife shall have made them suffer, I speak of women, whose parts shall have been all bruised, and so vilely treated and torn, as in some to lay the anus and vagina into one, besides their children being dismembered, some their arms or legs plucked off, others the whole body, the head being left behind in the uterus."

This is the language of a man-midwife himself, who candidly declaims against the errors of his fellow-practitioners, undoubtedly without designing that such their errors should be wrested into an objection to the practice of that art being committed to the men. Such a conclusion would in me be unfair, and a vain attempt to impose on the reader the laudable condemnation of an abuse, for an indiscriminate reproach to the whole set of men-midwives. This would however be but a kind of retaliative treatment of those, who, from the defective practice of the ignorant and unskilful midwives, of which if there was no more than one in the world, that one would be much too many, take the unjust handle of inveighing against midwives in general.

Even la Motte himself, who, as I have before with pleasure observed, was really as capable a man in the profession of midwifery as a man can be, at least to judge of him by his writings, has embraced every occasion of boasting the superiority of the men to the women in the exercise of midwifery. But while he taxes men of *scenes* that make one *shudder* with *horror*, the mistakes he imputes to the women, which are bad enough in all conscience, are not however of that atrocious nature, as those he relates of the men. Nay, with all his desire of under-rating the women, he falls into even pitiful contradictions. Let the reader himself decide on the following one.

Upon an article of practice, for which M. De la Motte blames the midwives, and what an article? Not such as he reproaches to the men-practitioners, murdering, maiming the women, or tearing their children limb from limb, but purely for their applying certain bandages to the belly of women after their lying-in, in order to keep that part smooth from wrinkles; this very author, I say, who allowed the Hôtel Dieu at Paris, where the manual function is wholly confined to women, to be the best school of midwifery in Europe, where he himself wished, and wished in vain, to be admitted to practice, and, in short, from the head-midwife, of which Madam de la Marche he himself probably learned all that was worth any thing in his practice, thus speaks of the midwives bred up in that hospital.

"This prerogative of having served apprentice in the Hôtel Dieu at Paris, is not for these women, an *indifferent* matter, for though they were to have no more than a *shadow* of *sense*, they are persuaded, that in setting themselves off with a *title* that does not render them more *capable*, they ought to be honored and respected above all others, which they would not fail of being, if they were to give some marks of sufficiency beyond what others can give[28]."

The nonsense of this objection of Mr. De la Motte is too glaring to need a comment. If an education in the best school of midwifery in Europe, does not give a woman a right to plead it for a title to reliance on her superior sufficiency, without any reason therefore to accuse her of vanity, what can give her a title?

But to return to M. De la Motte's sentiments on the practice of the men-midwives; it will easily be seen, that the horrors he objects to their practice, and of which he himself undoubtedly endeavoured to steer as clear as he could, were of a nature, without the least breach of candor, to suppose liable to repetitions wherever so false a doctrine and practice prevail as the substituting steel and iron-instruments, or "artificial hands" to natural ones.

Let us now see what Mr. De la Motte thinks of the use of the CROTCHET.

"When I settled in my province (says this author[29]) I found several ancient master-surgeons, who pretended to help the women in their difficult, or preternatural labors, solely with the use of the crotchet; without ever, in their life having made any *delivery*, but in that manner, and as soon as they had extracted the fœtus with their crotchet, they left the rest or the after-birth to be brought away by a woman, as they themselves knew nothing of the matter. When they were fetched to help a woman in labor, they took their crotchet, went to the woman, whom they put into posture, and whether the child presented the head, breech, arm or leg, whether it was dead or alive, a woman's having passed a day and a half in labor was cue more than enough for them to go to work with their crotchet."

The following extracts from the same Mr. De la Motte, may serve to confirm the foregoing observation.

---

[28] See La Motte, p. 646, of the quarto edition, Leyden.
[29] See La Motte, p. 262. lib. v. chap. 2.

"OBSERVATION 187. I was sent for to lay Madam de ——— about fifteen leagues from Valognes, the place of residence, and there was at the same time a surgeon of the town where I then was, who had been fetched to lay a woman that had been in labor from the day before, whose child presented the vertex: he, without further examination, put her into a convenient posture, and with his crotchet brought away the child at several pulls, with much pain and labor, and threw it under the bed, with the after-birth, in the most severe season of the year: after which, the operator hugged himself prodigiously, for having so happily accomplished so difficult a labor. Having rested a little, and just as he was going, a woman curious, bethought herself of seeing whether it was a boy or girl: she found the poor-child yet alive, though so mangled with the crotchet, and that after having remained, in this condition, an hour and a half, without its having been in the power of so violent an operation, or of the rigor of the weather to terminate a life which seemed to have held out against so many barbarities, only to reproach the detestable operator with the enormity of his crime. The child was christened and died soon after.

"REFLEXION. This is what may be called a cruel ignorance, &c."—To the which I add, that if this wretched operator had had the patience to wait some time, the child would in all probability have come naturally with any the least help of the hand at every throw of the mother: for she had not been over-time in labor, and the head was not, it seems, stuck in the passage.

"OBSERVATION 196, p. 274. I was desired to go to Cherbourg to lay a poor woman there, whom a surgeon and a man-midwife by a profession, belonging to that place, had given over ——— I found the woman in a condition hard to describe, with an arm and a leg of her child pulled off, and the remainder of the body left behind in the mother's womb. I put her into posture, and instantly delivered her of one child (it seems she went with twins) who had only and arm plucked off: I then sought out the other, whose leg had been torn away. Strange and fatal sight, which was seen by more than twenty women present, all ready to swear to the truth of this! I left the woman to their care, after having delivered her of the after-birth. She had been as much hurt as the children, of whom nothing remained in the uterus, by the care I took to evacuate it. I left the mother tolerably well considering her condition."

REFLEXION. This was the more surprizing, for that the first operator was an old practitioner, who had been an out-surgeon to the Hôtel Dieu above eight years, before M. De la Motte was apprentice there. Yet this man neither was sensible of the being twins in the case, nor had dexterity enough in the manual function. Here I ask, could the most ignorant midwife have, acquitted herself worse than this *man*?

"OBSERVATION 185. A tradesman's wife of Valognes being taken in labor sent for a midwife. A little while after her coming, the membranes burst, the waters were discharged, and the child presented an arm. The midwife required help. (Probably she might be one of the ignorant and unskilful ones) and two surgeons were sent for, who passed for being the most expert ones in the town. They begun with plucking off the arm that presented, though the child was *alive*. The other arm, as soon as they got hold of it, underwent the same fate. After which they struck the crotchet into a rib, which they brought away, then two, then three, and, at length, struck the crotchet into the back-bone, and pulled so cleverly together, that they brought the child away doubled up. The midwife delivered her of the afterbirth, and notwithstanding all this ill usage, the woman recovered; but it was a long while first."

REFLEXION. (Mr. De la Motte's own) Was there ever a crueler operation seen both for the mother and child; the first terribly torn, the other barbarously dismembered?

"OBSERVATION 186. The wife of a tallow-chandler of this town was taken in labor: the waters were discharged, after which an arm of the child presented. Help was sent for; one of the two operators (mentioned in the foregoing observation) came with his servant and crotchet. He began his operation, by plucking off the arm of this certainly live child, then, without further examination, he strikes the crotchet into its body, and pulled, without being able to bring away any thing. The master, whose strength was exhausted, made his pupil help him, and they both pulled as hard as they could: still nothing came, and I verily believe that the master would have called in some body else to his assistance, if the handle of the crotchet had been long enough, or that the poor woman had not given up the ghost under the cruel torments they made her suffer, to such a degree that they forced her to part with her life, sooner than with her child.

"REFLEXION. Here was a *delivery* in intention, but the execution had something horrid, and perfectly odious in it. I never could have imagined, that two men could have pulled in this manner, without dislocating the bones of the woman into whom the crotchet had been struck: for so it was shown to be, upon the body being opened, in which the child was found with an arm plucked off, entangled in the umbilical chord round its neck, without the least mark of the crotchet upon its body: too plain a proof this of the crotchet having been struck into the mother and not the child, and consequently of the little circumspection, not to say rage, with which the surgeon had acted upon the body of this unhappy creature: for surely it must be granted, that it could be no part of the child that could have resisted the terrible efforts made both by master and man, jointly to bring it away; and yet this was one of the BEST[30] operators in the country for HELPING women in labor.

"I could make a VOLUME of these histories, if they were good for any thing but to excite horror." Such is the witness born by M. De la Motte, as to the *ablest* men-midwives of his time, in all his province. Now in order to invalidate the conclusion, so natural to be drawn from so unexceptionable on attestation, against the superiority of the practice of the men to that of the women, will it be said, that the men-practitioners, in this country, are in general better educated than such operators as have been above shown? If so great a falsity should be advanced, let the reader himself reflect on what he may easily find to be the common method of training up of men-pupils in this art. I have in the first part of this work, stated some reasons for their insufficiency, both in study and practice; and the more this point is examined, the more clear will that undoubted truth appear, that if the ignorant midwives are, as they undoubted are, a great evil, they are even blessings in comparison to the generality of the men-practitioners, bred up with the help of artificial Dolls, pretty prints, or even of their personal visitation of those miserable wretches hired, or under the mask of charity, forced to undergo, from apprentices or pupils, so many inhuman tortures and outrages in vain.

It will also perhaps be said, as to the examples I have just produced from M. De la Motte, that since his time, that is to say, about the beginning of this century, that the art of midwifery has received so much improvement, as to cancel all impressions of fear from such examples. Yes! It has received improvement with a vengeance. If a vain endeavour to perfect instruments,

---

[30] If these *best* operators had been examined touching their opinion of midwives; they would most probably have told you, they were a parcel of poor insignificant ignorant creatures.

impossible to be perfected, or against common sense to suppose, even when perfected superior to skilful hands, are an improvement, then the art may be called improved. In the mean time, infinite is the mischief done by so many pretending operators, with each his bag of hard-ware at hand, his only proof of superiority to a woman, in practice, consisting in those instruments. Their negative damage is almost as great as their actual one. For by occasioning the men, and even ignorant midwives to trust to the calling in their help, the methods of predisposing of the women to parturition, the proper precautions, and actual manual function in the labor-pains, which is a point of the utmost importance, are at best but slightly and perfunctorily, consequently not sufficiently, performed, or perhaps wholly neglected. And why? Because the instruments, the *crotchet*, the *tire-tête*, the *forceps*, are considered as sure reserves to remedy such deficiencies. This, besides many other reasons, encourages the indolence, carelessness, and inattention of the men-practitioners, and even of the midwives, especially of those poor suborned creatures recommended by the men-practitioners, paid, as one may say in some sense; not to do their work so well, as that none should be left for their honorable patrons. Thence it has happened, that where an ignorant midwife has, through her unskilfulness, or for whatever other reason, been wanting in predisposing the passage, or lapsed the critical moments of the manual aid, so that she really is or pretends to be out of her depth, by the exigence being beyond her ability; the man-midwife is called in, who, with his instruments, forces that delivery, which might, if justice had been done to the patient, have proceeded in a natural way, with much less pain and danger. Be this remarked, without my speaking here of the extraordinary tortures and outrages, such as M. De la Motte himself has related. The woman then is, by the help of instruments, delivered by the man-midwife so called in. "If he had but staid a few minutes longer, both mother and child must have been lost". So believes the father of the child, so believes the mother, so believe most of the parties concerned, and what is more, sometimes so believes the man-midwife himself. Though the strict truth has been, that the greatest part of the pain the mother endured, and every appearance of danger, either to her or to her child, were positively owing to nothing but the negligence and mis-practice used, either by man or woman-practitioner, in reliance, if matters should come to the worst, on the supplemental aid or reparation of errors, by those miserable instruments, which constitute all the boasted improvements of an art, the true nicety and requisite accuracy of which they are so much more calculated to banish or destroy.

I have however quoted the foregoing examples from M. De la Motte.

First, Because that he himself being a man-midwife, and greatly partial to the practice being best in the hands of men, his attestation must be the less suspicious: but especially, because he was a professed enemy to instruments, and adhered as closely as Nature would allow him, to the imitation of those midwives from whom he had received all his *knowledge*, and abused them afterwards for their *ignorance*, as if their communication to him of their knowledge could not have been, without leaving themselves wholly destitute of it to enrich him.

Secondly, Because, the stories which he relates upon his own knowledge, leaving me the fairest room to infer the necessary repetition of the like tragical wents wherever instruments are admitted, it became less invidious to specify them, than incidents of the like nature here: especially, I say here, in London, or in England, where the use of those instruments grows every day more and more rise, and must consequently furnish the more examples of pain, destruction and danger caused by them to the women, weak or prejudice-ridden enough to prefer the men to the women-practitioners.

Both Charity then and Prudence prescribe to me the not pointing out particular persons to whom I could impute mis-practice. If any one will affect to treat this suppression as not owing thereto, but purely to an impossibility of specifying cases of that sort, and of proving them; I appeal to the candid reader, whether the nature of the charge considered, such a specification can be expected from me, since, from the examples I have produced, I pretend to infer no more than a probability, the grounds of which I submit to himself, of the repetition of the like acts from the same, or even from increasing the same practice.

It would not perhaps be otherwise impossible to give some instances. For example, I could expand a hint before given, of a man-midwife of this town, who passes for eminent in his profession, and who not above five years ago, was called to deliver a woman in labor, whose child presented an arm. This practitioner, instead of scarching out for the feet, to extract this fœtus, that was quite alive, first plucks off one arm, then another, then, at length, gives over the job, and left the poor mother in this condition, who was forced to have recourse to a midwife to finish the delivery.

More than one operator, as I have before observed, in very natural deliveries, instead of bringing away the after-birth, tore out the body of the uterus; for all their boasted anatomy.

Another gentleman-midwife delivered a woman of a fine child, or rather received it, for it came naturally and easily. Upon which, he took it into his head that he would not deliver her of the after-birth, proposing to defer this work till next day. And so he would have done, if he had not casually met with a less senseless practitioner, who represented to him the danger to which, by so doing, he exposed the poor patient he had left, and advised him to go back as fast as he could to deliver her.[31]

I have myself been not a little surprized at hearing lately some ladies mention, with much approbation, the inimitable complaisance of certain gentlemen-midwives, who have the patience, as they call it, to wait five, six, seven hours by the clock, before they deliver of the after-birth after the issue of the child, and that out of tenderness to the patients, who, as they say, would be sadly off, if they fell into hands more quick and expeditious.

But while I am thus taking notice of the errors of practice in the men-practitioners, it may be objected to me, that I deal unfairly with my reader.

First, In not furnishing instances of male-practice of the midwives.

Secondly, That whereas I have confessed the incapacity of some of the midwives, without allowing inferences from them against all the professors of the art who are of the female sex, I ought to make the same equitable allowance as to the men-practitioners, and not condemn all for the sake of those unsufficient ones, which the capable ones themselves candidly condemn, witness among others, M. De la Motte.

Now, as to my omitting such a specification of instances of mis-practice in my own sex, it is neither from partiality, nor affectation, that this omission of mine proceeds. For could any one be so weak as retaliatively to state cases, in the manner I have done, of mis-practice of some midwives; nothing could be

---

[31] Dr. Smellie seems to countenance this practice, where he says, p. 232. "*We have already observed, (p. 229) that if there is no danger from a flooding, the woman may be allowed to rest a little, in order to recover from the fatigue she has undergone, and that the uterus may in contracting have time to squeeze and separate the placenta from its inner surface.*"

more superfluous, nor less to the purpose. My confession, my lamentation, that there are but too many ignorant midwives, palpably obviate the necessity of proving what is granted. The public would be very little the better for a truth, with which it cannot but be too well acquainted, that there are ignorant midwives, and insufficient men-practitioners. The truth then, for which I contend, is, that the faults of the midwives, however it may be wished that they could be prevented, are, comparatively speaking, neither so likely to exist in Nature, nor of that horrid, atrocious kind, that are to be found in the practice of the men-practitioners or instrumentarians. There is nothing among the midwives of the puncturing, tearing with cold pinchers, maiming, mangling, pulling limb from limb, disabling, as must be inseparable in a greater or less degree from the use of those iron and steel-instruments, which are so often and so unnecessarily employed.

As to the second objection, of my not making any distinction of the capable from the incapable men-practitioners. The reason of that is obvious. It results from the fairest comparison of the two sexes, in respect to midwifery, independent of any such examples as have been produced against any particular individuals of that profession in the men. Nature has so favored the midwives, that among them the bad ones are evidently an exception to the general rule, of the fitness of that sex for the art: whereas among men, the bad practitioners are, and must for ever be, the general rule, and the good ones the exception, if so it is, that, in Nature, there can be such an exception: he that makes a practice of using instruments can hardly be one.

Nothing however will more conduce to establish the natural disqualification of the men for this art, than a fair consideration of that capitally essential branch of it, the ART of TOUCHING, in order to ascertain the state of pregnant women, and the difficulties so necessary to be foreknown in order to be lessened or avoided. On due prevention often depends the saving the life of both mother and child; it cannot then be thought a digression, that I transiently give a summary account of this great light or guidance to that prevention, even though this work is nothing of a regular treatise of the art.

OF TOUCHING.

Conducively to a just idea of touching, there should be a just foundation laid of a competent knowledge of the fabric of the sexual parts, of the conformation of the *pelvis*, and of the bones which constitute it. There requires no depth of anatomy to know, in general, that the *pelvis* is composed of that part of the backbone called the *os sacrum*, terminated at the bottom by the *coccyx*, of the *ilia*, and the *os pubis*. In the cavity formed by the assemblage of these bones is the *uterus*, suspended between the bladder and the *intestinum rectum*, by four ligaments called broad and round. The two broad ones are a production of the *peritonœum*, on the side of the *vertebræ*, and terminate on each side of the uterus near the fallopian tubes. The round issue on the side of the *fundus uteri*, immediately under the tubes, and from thence passing through the *peritonœum*, and crossing the muscles of the hypogastrium, are inserted at the pubis and common membrane or integument of the forepart of the thighs. I pretend here nothing further, than to give a summary sketch of these parts, a more particularized one being here needless. Suffize it to observe, that no good midwife can be without a proper and distinct conception of their position and conformation, not only for touching, but for operating with success.

Touching, in the terms of art, consists in the introduction of one or two fingers into the vagina, and thereby into the orifice of the uterus of the person, whose state or situation requires to be known. There scarcely needs admonishing on this occasion, a midwife, of the due care of her hands, being properly prepared and guarded from the least danger of hurting. Such a precaution recommends itself.

The touch then is the most nice and essential point of the art of midwifery. Nor to acquire a sufficient degree of accuracy in it, can there be too much pains taken, considering how much depends on it. Midwives only of great practice, or lying-in hospitals, where there is full liberty for the young female practitioners to make observations, can render it familiar to the learner. I presume I may take for granted, that such a practical study is not extremely decent, nor proper for young lads. And yet, at their season of life it is, that this study should be begun, if but to give expertness the necessary time to attain, through habit, its full growth, against the age of exercising the manual function. It must surely be rather too late, for a man to commence his course of touching at the age of practising; as it must be too soon, at a season of life, where his capital end of *touching* will probably not be the acquisition of the science. At whose expence then must the rudiments of a man's study of this branch of the art be? Surely at that of the unfortunate women, subjected to the annoyance of such nauseous and profitless visitation. In short, this is ONE of the points of the art, from the nature of which it may fairly, and without implication of contradiction, be pronounced, that the greatest anatomist in Europe may nevertheless be a very indifferent, not to say a miserable man-midwife: or even that a very indifferent anatomist may for all that be an excellent manual practitioner.

A midwife, duly qualified by Nature and art, with a shreudness and delicacy of the touch, is, when requisite, capable of giving, in virtue thereof, a just account of a woman's condition. She is enabled to make faithful reports to the physician, and inform him of the needful concerning the state of his patient, where any co-incidence of pregnancy sollicits his attention. By the same means she can distinguish the true labor-pains from the false ones; and when the term of delivery is at hand, it may, by the touch, be discerned, whether the labor will be easy or hard, whether the fœtus is well or ill situated. With other precognitions, highly necessary for our taking proper measures both obviative and actual.

I say necessary, because it is from this practice of touching that we draw our prognostics, both for the predisposition of the passage, in order to save pain by proper anticipation, and to smooth or facilitate a happy delivery. It is then the touch that serves us for a guide, and certifies to us the situation of the uterus, its rectitude or its obliquity, as well as what part of the fœtus presents.

It is in short by the information we receive from the touch, that we are enabled in good time to remedy, or at least to lessen all the obstacles: so that by the very same means, by which we obviate any necessity of recourse to instruments, we at the same time alleviate the pains and sufferings of the party: which one would think no inconsiderable advantage of the female over the male practice, which last is so constitutionally more rough and more violent.

Such is the capital importance of the TOUCH, undeniable, I presume even by the men-practitioners. But will any of the he-midwives then, with those special delicate soft hands of theirs, and their long taper pretty fingers, pretend to vye with the women in the exquisite sense or faculty of the touch, with which Nature herself has so palpably indowed and qualified them for the necessary shreudness of discernment, that in them it can scarcely be deemed an acquisition of art? If the encroachments however of the male-practitioners proceed, under color of their vast superiority, I should not be surprized at seeing, ere long, a grave set of grey-bearded gentlemen-midwives impannelled in lieu of a jury of matrons, on a female convict pleading her belly. What can hinder the redress of such a grievance, as the law has authorized for so many ages, but the object not being one of a pecuniary enough interest to tempt the men to interfere in it? They would be in the wrong however not to apply for the office, since it would not be one of the least innocent occasions for them to improve their hand in the mistery of *touching*.

But let them pretend what they will, so great is the advantage, so liberal of her gift has Nature been to women, in that aptitude of theirs, which may be termed a knack of touching, that the hand of a true midwife will, at the deriving of indications from the report of its touch, beat the most scientific head of a man-practitioner, though stuffed never so full with Greek and Latin. Yes, an ignorant midwife, without perhaps anatomy enough to know where the *pineal gland* is, or without so much as having heard the name of the *ossa innominata*, and with purely her expertness, and with that sort of knowledge she has at her fingers ends, will give you a more useful and practical account of matters, as they go, where it is sometimes so infinitely important to know how they go, than the most learned anatomist that ever dissected a corpse, brandished a forceps, stuck a crotchet into a child's brain-pan, or tore open a living woman.

Upon this point of touching there occurs a consideration, on which I have before just transiently touched, and beg leave, for the sake of its importance, to give it some expansion.

In my objection to a man's practising this branch of art, TOUCHING, I wave here the natural repugnance all the parties must have to it, even the man-midwife himself, on any footing but of that of interest, allowing an exclusion of any libertine design, I wave especially the argument against it, from its being a kind of invasion of a husband's incommunicable prerogative; I even wave the breach of modesty, I suppose all this to be answered by the plea of superior safety, however false and imaginary that plea may be. But surely it will be allowed me to pity the unfortunate condition of a woman, subjected to so disagreeable a visitation; a visitation which, instead of being performed in the gentle, congenial, and especially, as to the end, satisfactory manner, of which the women alone are capable, must furnish a scene, not only unprofitable, disgustfully coarse, and even ridiculous, but also most probably a very painful. Figure to yourself that respectable personage a He-midwife, quite as grave and solemn as you please, with a look composed to all that "DELICACY *of* DECORUM," recommended by Dr. Smellie, and so suitable to the high DIGNITY of the *office* he is undertaking of *touching* the unhappy woman, subjected to his pretentions of useful discovery by it. What must not parts, which dispute exquisiteness of sensibility with the eye itself, suffer from hands, naturally none of the softest, and perhaps callous with handling iron and steel instruments, from some hands, in short, scarce less hard than the instruments themselves, boisterously grabbling and rummaging for such nice indications, as their want of fineness in the touch must for ever refuse them? what if they may possibly, by such coarse *touching*, find some common, obvious signs presenting themselves, so that the grossest touch cannot escape distinguishing them; does it therefore follow, that the nicer points, on which so much may depend for preparatory disposal, will not escape hands, scarce not less disqualified for the necessary discernment, than a midwife's if she had gloves on? In the mean while, what torture must not the poor woman endure, in every sense, from the wounds of modesty, and even of her person? and for what? that the doctor may, with a significant nod, or silent shrug, give himself the false air of being satisfied about what he was pretending to look for; or, if he speaks, come off with some jargon, only the more respectfully received by the patient, for its neither being common sense, nor intelligible to her; or perhaps, if he has any by-ends in view, or is a man of gallantry, here is a fine occasion for his placing a compliment. But for any essential advantage to her, from such a quackery of painful perquisition, she need not expect it. The infinitely important service of predisposing the passages, and of obviating difficulties, to be only ascertained by that faculty of touching, is palpably and peculiarly appropriated by Nature to the women only; and it is from them alone that a woman must, naturally and truly speaking, be the least shocked at receiving such service. Whereas in being *touched* by a man, besides, I once more say, besides the revoltingness of Nature, and the protest of female modesty against it, besides the pain inseparable from it, besides even its insufficiency; the safety of the woman is destroyed to the very foundations, by the negation of due foreknowledge and proper disposal, against the actual crisis of danger or the real labor-pains, the mitigation of which, and facilitating the delivery, depend so much on the *accuracy* of the *touch*.

Whoever then will but consider that greater aptitude of organization in the women for fineness of that sense of touching, will allow, that I beg no question, when I aver, proverbially, but truly speaking, that if one hundred points of qualification were requisite to constitute this capital faculty of TOUCHING, a midwife already possesses, in the but being a woman, ninety-nine of them, the sure and certain gift of Nature: and the remaining one from Art, may with great ease, with a little instruction and experience, be acquired. Whereas, the He-midwife, not only, as not being a woman, wants the whole ninety-nine, but can never receive the hundredth at the hands of Art, but in so imperfect a degree, that his trusting it will make it worse to the unfortunate woman that shall trust him, than if he was wholly without it. I might perhaps, not without reason, extend this allegation of the superiority of the female sex over the male in this point, and in the same proportion, to the whole of the manual function, but that I am more afraid of exaggerating, than even of falling short of the truth.

Surely then, one might imagine, that the parties principally concerned in liquidating this difference for the government of their decision, on a point of such capital importance, would not do amiss to consider it, before they suffer themselves to be imposed upon in the manner they are by the men-pretenders to a purely female office. An imposition so very gross, that instead of answering the end of those on whom it passes, that of greater safety, only encreases the dreaded danger. And most assuredly, the women who subject themselves to it, do so, if with no scandal to their modesty at least to their understanding; for being sunk to so low a degree of cheapness, as even to purchase, with a sort of prostitution, innocent let it be, it is still a prostitution, after which money is a consideration beneath mention, and to purchase what? danger to their own life, danger to that of the pretious burthen within them, and, at the very least, an increase of bodily pain to themselves.

Mr. De la Motte, in his 188th OBSERVATION, p. 265, *Leyden ed.* makes an animadversion upon a midwife's *touching* a patient, which, unless he was

141

induced to it by that spirit of injustice to midwives in general, against which injustice all his usual candor is sometimes not proof, would persuade me, that he was more ignorant of the nature and ends of *touching*, than what his works show him to have been in other parts of the profession.

In that OBSERVATION he gives you the case of a woman in labor, to whom he was called, whose membranes a midwife had prematurely broke, whom she had actually over-fatigued with making her too often shift her posture, and also with incessant and reiterated TOUCHINGS (*attouchemens qu'elle reiteroit sans relâche*) and all this, from a principle of avarice, in order to make the quicker riddance, for the sake of attending a richer patient, where she expected greater gain; "as if (says Mr. De la Motte, in words that ought to be engraved in every practitioner's heart) a poor woman was more to be neglected than a wealthy one, in the presence of a God who judges all our actions."

For my quoting this case, especially as it regards the point of TOUCHING now under discussion, my reason, from the considerations to which it will give rise in the reader's own mind, will probably appear so satisfactory to him, that he will easily absolve me of any charge of digression.

As to the midwife's bringing on the premature discharge of the waters, if the fact was true: it was very blameable practice. It is a practice that all capable midwives reprove and forbid, as it is robbing the part of the most natural and necessary lubrication for facilitating the launch in due time of the fœtus. I have been assured, with what truth I cannot well warrant, that the men-practitioners are commonly much too precipitate in the breaking of the membranes. Be the practitioners then of what sex they may, such practice is bad.

But, as to the motive M. De la Motte attributes to the midwife, of avarice for such a procedure, I should heartily join with him in condemning her, if the mention he makes of the REITERATED TOUCHINGS did not make me suspect not his sincerity but his knowledge. If the poor midwife had been to write the case, I have the charity to think she could, with truth, have given a better a reason for her practice than suggestion of avarice. At the worst, however, so criminal a spring of action in such a conjuncture, could only be personal to herself, not affect the midwives in general. Mr. De la Motte himself would own this, who, as the reader may see p.286, does not spare the men-practitioners on this head, without meaning, that he or his fraternity should be involved in any sinister inference from thence. And, indeed, I should have a right to laugh at men-practitioners reproaching the midwives with interestedness. I fancy I can have few readers so ignorant, as not to know by which of the two sexes the greater fees are expected; which sex, in short, looks the most out of humor, when those same fees do not amount to the practitioner's idea of the DECORUM of his "DIGNITY."

But let the pass. I come now to the great point of the TOUCHINGS complained of by M. De la Motte, and I sincerely believe unjustly complained of. My cause of such belief is this: I am well grounded in my averring, that in many labors much depends on the rectification of things, (this will be hereafter more at large explained) by the act of touching, not only reiterated, but sometimes even not to be discontinued for hours together. And these *touchings* are so far from fatiguing, or vexing the patient, that they often prove her greatest relief from pain, and even preservation from danger, by the facilitation they procure to the issue of the fœtus, that is to say, if they are skilfully managed.

I have myself known women in pain, and even before their labor-pains came on, find, or imagine they found, a mitigation of their complaints, by the simple application of the midwife's hand; gently chasing or stroaking them: a mitigation which, I presume, they would have been ashamed to ask, if they had been weak enough to expect it, from the delicate fist of a great-horse-godmother of a he-midwife, however softened his figure might be by his pocket-night-gown being of flowered callico, or his cap of office tied with pink and silver ribbons; for I presume he would scarce, against Dr. Smellie's express authority, go about a function of this nature in a full-suit, and a tie-wig.

I am also the more ready to believe, that these same *touchings*, with which M. De la Motte, finds fault had in this case been really of service, since he confesses, he found the child *"well situated, and FAR ADVANCED in the passage"*; and withal offers no reason to think, but that it was so *far advanced* from the *touchings*, not in spite of the *touchings*.

We shall now see what followed. Mr. De la Motte, that despiser of midwives; Mr. De la Motte, who so consistently regretted his not being admitted to the Hôtel Dieu at Paris, and accuses the women, educated at that Hospital, of vanity, for valuing themselves on that education, behaved himself on this occasion, as indeed his merit was that on most occasions he did so, like a true good midwife: he found things *far advanced* enough, for him to leave the rest very wisely to Nature, and so he did. The consequence of which was, that the patient was soon delivered of a fine boy, and both mother and child did well.

Such was the result of Mr. De la Motte's true midwifely proceeding. But what would an instrumentarian have probably done? One of those, I say, who, as to all the boasted improvement of the obstetrical art, produce the stupendous inventions of those surely rather weapons of death, than of life, which Dr. Smellie calls his REINFORCEMENTS, and is so good as "*principally*" to recommend, "*namely the small forceps, blunt hook, scissors, and curve crotchets*" the unenviable privilege of using which blessed substitutes to the soft fingers of women, being supposed inherent to the men by right of superiority of skill, has so greatly IMPROVED the art of midwifery, and thinned the number of good midwives, by exploding their so much less painful, and certainly more safe method of practice, both for mother and child? For after all, what can such instruments be expected to do, but, instead of improving the art, to multiply murders? if this should appear too severe, hear what Mr. De la Motte himself says to the very case in point: to this very case, in which himself, I repeat it, did no more than play the part of the good midwife, and was only the more commendable for doing so.

"If the operator of the place had been called, he would DOUBTLESS have proceeded in this delivery, as he had done in the other (see p. 292.) that is to say, he would have *quickly* dispatched it with his *crotchet*: but on the contrary, if he had had any experience, he would have conducted the other delivery as I did this, and thereby have exempted himself from the reproach he must have made to himself, for having killed a poor woman in the most *cruel* manner."

Happy! thrice happy it is for the midwives, that, at least, if avarice should tempt any of them to the injustice of hurrying a poor patient's delivery, in order to attend a rich one; a circumstance which, I fancy however, does not more often occur to the female than to the male-practitioners; the woman cannot, at least, use towards precipitating such deliveries means so violent as the men. They appear only in guise of peaceable simple seconds to Nature: the men take the field, armed as combatants against her. The women can but prematurate things by excitation of the hand; they may be guilty of reprehensible negligence, they may be over curious in their bandages, by way of smoothing wrinkles after delivery; in short, they may commit many faults, which I am far from justifying, or even extenuating; but at the very worst, I defy them to equal the instrumentarians in mischief; nor can their practice abound with those horrors, of which a man-midwife tells us he could furnish VOLUMES (p. 298.) horrors which must be so greatly multiplied since his time, as the recourse to instruments is more than ever pursued, in practice, though so fallaciously disowned in the theory; under which disavowal the gentlemen midwives figuratively conceal their bag of hardware, just as Dr. Smellie directs them literally to do in their visits to patients.

But to resume the subject of TOUCHING, I am to observe, that among its essential services on many occasions, both during the pregnancy, and in the actual labor-pains, there is one case, which, for its frequency and importance, deserves a separate consideration: it is that of the obliquity of the uterus, of which touching not only serves to inform, but to rectify it. I shall therefore dedicate a section to the treating OF IT.

OF THE OBLIQUITY OF THE UTERUS.

By the obliquity of the uterus I mean its untoward situation. For either the uterus preserves its natural direction, or does not preserve it. Where the uterus preserves it, I call it well placed: the point of it is turned directly to the cavity of the pelvis, and the *fundus uteri* is suspended in the space between the umbilical region and the vertebræ: if the uterus does not preserve its natural direction, if it inclines too much forwards, backwards, or towards either the right or the left side, I call it oblique, or untowardly placed. All the other situations of the uterus are rediculble to these four, from which they differ no otherwise than as its line that should naturally be perpendicular to that of the vagina deviates more or less from it towards any of them. It is from this obliquity, greater or less, that proceeds, by much the most often, the greater or the less difficulty of the lyings-in.

It would be superfluous here to analise all the causes of such obliquity, because, being mostly natural ones, there is no preventing them. But there are some causes of it, or at least, that appear to me to be sometimes the causes of it, that it cannot be improper for me to premise here, for precaution-sake.

I have then some reason to think, that both here and in Holland the stays contribute much to the obliquity of the uterus. For though women, during their pregnancy, may perhaps wear them looser than at other times; yet their natural hardness pressing on the belly, with the stiff whalebones, always too many if there are any at all, cramp the fœtus and the womb, to which the stays too often give a bid situation, according to their motion or swagging more to one side than to the other, in their state of looseness; and if they were laced tighter, that would be yet more dangerous.

I could wish then, that women with child would either content themselves with wearing a bodice only, or stays without any whalebone, but at the back just to serve the loins, and even those not to come so low down as I have seen some. The obliquity of the uterus is much rarer in France than it is here, for which I cannot account otherwise, than from the women there avoiding any prejudice from their stays, during their pregnancy. There is another cause, as I apprehend it, of the lateral byass, which is the lying too constantly on either side, whence the uterus contracts a habit of inclination to that side. The probability of such an effect I submit to the anatomists, as I speak here only conjecturally, and not with the presumption of certainty.

The obliquity of the uterus may be discerned from the difficulty there will be, in touching, to come at its orifice. And it is by touching alone that you can hope to discover which way its deviation points, whether it is placed too high towards the *os pubis*, too much turned towards the curve of the vertebræ, or in a lateral direction, towards either the right or left *ilion*. But which ever way that mis-direction points, the difficulty of the delivery is proportionable to the degree of it: and the skill and knowledge of the midwife in not only the reduction, but the keeping of the uterus to its due position, till the delivery is accomplished, form one of those principal branches of the art, for which the gentlemen-midwives must be naturally so unfit.

There are very few authors who have treated of this obliquity of the uterus. Some do not mention it at all, others speak of it, but so slightly as to escape attention.

Dr. Smellie in his enumeration of the cases, by which laborious labors are occasioned, which he ranges under seven heads, has intirely omitted this case of obliquity. He has bestowed indeed a whole chapter on the distortion of the pelvis, a case I take to be comparatively infinitely rarer than an obliquity of the

146

uterus. He might as well suppose a frequent vitious conformation of the cheek-bones, as of those that form the pelvis: which, were it so, must necessarily imply a constant recurrence of hard labors in the same woman, which is not often the case. Whereas the liableness of the uterus to an obliquity from various accidents, principally accounts for the easiness of one labor in a woman, being no argument for her not having a hard one in future, of convertibly. I dare aver then, that in the course of my practice, which is not the least extensive one, this very case of obliquity has occurred to me oftener than all the others put together, and indeed caused me the most pain to remedy or conquer. Why then such an omission by these writers? I cannot conceive, unless that they were aware of the consequence, obvious to be drawn from thence, that women, by the superior fitness of their hands, must be the properest to apply the topical remedy; and that their iron and steel instruments could not so well be set to work in such a case, at least in due time. This is absolutely so true, that in the case of this very obliquity, which occasions most of the very lingering labors, for which the midwives, who have hot preventively exerted themselves to reduce it, and thereby to clear the passage for the fœtus, have no remedy but patience; those very lingering labors, I say, which shall have thus arisen from the want of skill or prevention, furnish the men-practitioners with a pretence to dispatch them with their instruments. Thus they, often murderously for the child, and injuriously to the mother, terminate many a delivery, which a gentle and constant reduction of the uterus would have so much more safely and less painfully accomplished. And how accomplished? evidently not by any violence to Nature, but purely by redressing the wrong she is in, oftenest not by her own fault, but by some adventitious cause, in which she has been rather a passive sufferer than originally herself deficient. A justice this of distinction too often refused her, and from which too many errors of practice arise, perhaps in more cases than this.

However, this is certain, that this case of the obliquity of the uterus deserves much more notice and attention than have been paid to it. It is one of the most important difficulties of the art.

He who treats the most at large of this matter is Daventer, who, I have strong reasons for believing, first took the hint from some midwife: but a hint, which the usual imperfection of the manual function in men hindered him from duly improving. For in the way he sets forth the different inclinations of the uterus, and the methods of rectifying them, instead of throwing a practical light upon the subject, he has obscured it with errors, absurdities, and repetitions without number or excuse.

But that I may not appear to treat this author dogmatically, and especially as he furnishes me with an occasion of further elucidating a point of such great importance to the art of which I am treating, I must here intreat the attention of those readers, especially who deign to peruse me rather in the search of useful truth, than of amusement, of which indeed so serious a matter is so little susceptible.

Let us then examine some of Daventer's methods of practice, so unconsequential to so just a theory as that of the mis-direction incident to the uterus.

Daventer, chap xlvi. p. 288, French edition, treating of the rectification of an obliquity of the uterus fallen forwards, goes on thus. "When the membrane is broke, and the vertex of the head partly come forth, there is no longer occasion to support, as before, the orifice of the uterus. It should be let fall with the head beyond the curvature of the os sacrum. The head will make its way much more easily than if it was still wrapped up in the uterus (indeed!) Now to make the fœtus come forth, the midwife must, as she did at the beginning, employ both her hands; the one internally applied, the other externally; but take care so to do judiciously. Neither must she wait till the labor-pains are over, before she sets her hands to work, as I have just before observed. On the contrary, it is in the time of the throws that she must operate, and when they are on the decline, terminate the delivery. The midwife therefore should not barely content herself with watching the time of the pains, but should also admonish, at every one of them, her patient to second them with all her strength, in order that the child may advance the more under their stronger protrusion. During which, the midwife having her hand in the vagina, the back turned towards the rectum is to advance the tip of her fingers, the most she can, under the head of the child, taking care however not to over-press them; and in this posture, she is to keep her hands unmoveable, till she feels the labor-pains come on. The other hand she is to put on the hypogastrium, nearly over the place answering to the fundus uteri; and when the pains shall begin, she is to give her hands such action, that that which is in the vagina shall push back the coccyx, and the other applied externally shall push up gently the fundus uteri, and at the same time determine its orifice towards the pelvis. I say gently. But this is to be understood of the beginning of the throws, for in proportion as they increase, the midwife must press the harder.

Care must, in the mean time, be taken, that the pression made on the belly must not be too violent but *very* moderate: whereas that made on the coccyx must be with the midwife's whole strength, with this attention however, *first*, that this great effort must not be made but when the force of the throws obliges the woman strongly to contract the muscles of the hypogastrium, and must cease with those throws. *Secondly*, that the hand must be laid flat on the coccyx, not with the fingers half-bent, least the joints should hurt the woman. *Thirdly*, that the hand may be as much expanded as possible, that the pression may be equal on all parts. Observing these three conditions, the midwife may employ her *whole* strength, without *fear* of doing any harm to the woman. On the contrary, she will greatly relieve her."

To the which I have to say, that I should greatly pity a woman that should fall under the hands of a woman that should receive such directions from Monsieur l'Accoucheur, and much more yet, if she was to be under his. A midwife to operate thus! with one hand in and the other out, over the lower part of the belly, "gently" says Daventer, and yet stronger in proportion as the throws increase: and a little after he says, this pression on the belly must not be too violent, but *very* moderate. I confess, I do not understand, but that may be my fault, how a pression can be stronger and stronger as the pains increase, without ceasing to be gentle or very moderate.

Besides; as to the pression of the midwife's hand on the coccyx of the patient, so violent as he advises it, with the whole strength of the midwife, can this be executed without causing to the vagina or rectum a contusion, very capable of bringing on a gangrene, of causing a mortification, or, in short, the laceration of the frænum labiorum, whatever he may say to the contrary?

I observe, by the way, that in this very chapter Daventer supposes the heads of children breaking themselves, sometimes against the os pubis, or the vertebræ, as if these were bare bones, at least he is to me, in these points, unintelligible.

He goes on to object, that if, through ignorance, Nature has been so far left to herself, that the point of the uterus should be fallen into the pelvis, that its orifice, and the head of the child, should be fallen into the lower curve of the *os sacrum*, that the membrane should be broke, and the child's head a little discovered, and withal, the woman's strength much exhausted,

"To change, (says Daventer) this situation, thus you must proceed. The woman must rest upon her knees and elbows, with her head low. And what (adds he) determines the placing a woman in this posture, is, that the weight of the uterus may impel it to the side of the diaphragm, and consequently withdraw it from the sinuosity of the coccyx."

To me it appears impossible, that a woman, whose strength shall have been exhausted, or but much diminished, can put herself into such a posture, which could only serve to make her lose any little strength she might have left.

At the end of the said chap. xlvi. Daventer concludes in the following terms.

"However, to say the truth, of whatever kind the obliquity of the uterus may be, I hold, that the safest, the easiest, and the least painful expedient, is the footling-extraction of the child, from the very beginning of the labor, before or immediately after the discharge of the waters, as soon as one can be assured that the pains the woman feels are the labor-pains. If this method should be followed, which I hope (adds he) it will one day be, it would preserve an incredible number of women and children, the unhappy victims of a contrary practice."

Here I must confess the shallowness of my understanding. Such a reasoning as Daventer's in this case passes my conception. He allows, that in all the obliquities of the uterus, it is extremely difficult to find the orifice, to come at it, and to introduce the fingers into it: nay, he owns, that it is not without a great deal of trouble, that you can get to touch but the surface of that orifice; and after that confession, he tells you very gravely that, in such cases, you must deliver the child by the feet, in the very beginning of the labor, before even the discharge of the waters, or at least soon after.

Ought then the translator of Daventer, who is at the same time his apologist, in good conscience, boast so much the discoveries of this author upon the obliquity of the uterus? is it possible for common sense to give the approbation that he does to those easiest, safest, and least painful methods, that he recommends for relieving the mother and child in those cases of obliquity?

I am then too much prepared to be surprized, in the chapter following that from which I have quoted, to find him, where treating of an uterus too much inclined towards the vertebræ, not scruple to reason as follows.

150

"But if the child is too much compressed, or has a head over large, so that it is not without much difficulty to the midwife, and pain to the woman, that it can be hoped to bring the child into the pelvis, a state of things which does not unseldom happen, I judge that, to prevent the danger, the best method is the footling-extraction. But (adds our author by way of reflexion) this work is more *befitting* a *man* than a *woman*, unless she has a *quick* judgment, and an *alert* hand: a man-midwife should therefore be called (*Doubtless!*) and he must lay his account with having work enough, for it is not without a great deal of trouble and difficulty, that he will accomplish the turning the child, and that for *three* reasons.

"The First. Commonly, the orifice of the uterus in this situation is but little open: it must be *violently* dilated, that is to say, in *forcing* Nature, or *doing violence* to her: Yet this must be done slowly, for too much precipitation would cause to the woman *very acute pains*. (*To be sure, a slow violence would not hurt her.*)

"Reason the Second. It is not more easy to penetrate to the bottom of the uterus, of which the orifice already, narrow as it must be, is moreover occupied by the head of the child, than to open the orifice. No wonder then, that so much trouble and patience should be required to get at the child's feet.

"Thirdly, It will be found, that the distance there is between the orifice of the vagina to the bottom of the uterus, must render the *man-midwife's* work so much the more difficult for the sinuosity of it, and his being forced to operate in a part so narrow and close, and in which the hand is much cramped for room. It is obvious to sense, that a place so oblique and streight must deny the liberty of passage."

The advice which Daventer gives here of extracting the child by the feet in the case he supposes, and, for that purpose, violently to dilate the orifice of the uterus, appears to my weak mind such mad, such frantic doctrine, as to be beneath refutation. The bare recital of his own reasons, and of the difficulties there are to surmount, which he himself confesses, abundantly demonstrate the impossibility and absurdity of the method he proposes.

But after taking the liberty of dissenting from that celebrated man-midwife in cases of obliquity, as to the practical part, which I take indeed to be his *own* discovery, it is but just I should offer what I conceive to be the true midwife's practice, for terminating happily the labor of a woman in the case of obliquity of the uterus: submitting the same to better judgment.

All the deflexions or byasses of the uterus, whatever they are, are to be known by the touch. An expert and knowing hand will never fail of ascertaining the discovery of them. I say, an expert and knowing hand, for without an exact knowledge of the figure of the whole pelvis, the situation of the bladder, of the rectum, the vagina, and the uterus, before and after pregnancy, the situation of the orifice with respect to the pelvis, there is no distinguishing for example, an over-elevated orifice from one too low, nor a direct from an oblique one. In vain would one conceive clearly what those terms signify, or have some knowledge of the distinctive parts of the female sex, without one has at the same time sufficient experience, and fineness of sense in the touching part. Without these qualifications there is no proceeding but darkling, and in danger of deception.

The orifice of the uterus is always diamatrically opposite to the fundus of it. When then you know what the situation of the orifice of the uterus is, when in its due place, you may, if well versed in *touching*, calculate any aberration from the right line, and by the situation of the orifice giving that of the fundus, know how the rest is disposed.

When, by *touching*, I perceive, there is an obliquity of the uterus in the case, in the proper time, I desire the patient to lay on her back, and introducing my singer, endeavour to come at the orifice of the uterus. Upon getting hold of it, I support it so long as the labor-throw continues, and I take care the child should not engage itself too much.

I am obliged, with my hand, continually to repeat this service; and after resting a little from the fatigue, whenever I can snatch a moment safely for such relaxation, I re-introduce my finger, as before, in order to prevent the pains, and hinder the orifice from falling, that is to say, from sinking, so as to turn too much backwards, or from rising too high, or, in short, from deviating towards the right or the left, according to the circumstances or kinds of inclination that may present themselves. I also take great care, that the child may not engage itself too far under the os pubis. I do not discontinue these cares, these attentions, until, whatever assiduity, length of time, or trouble it may cost me, I shall have arrived at rectifying the wrong direction, by thus constantly supporting the internal orifice, till, in short, I have brought it, little by little, to turn and come directly on a line with the external orifice. By this management of the hand, I procure the child a fair opening, and its falling forward, without being wrapped up or embarrassed in the uterus.

And yet, in certain cases of obliquity I sometimes find so great an inversion of order, such an intanglement, that the child presents itself in the vagina with the body of the uterus covering it wholly, and by its volume totally impeding the coming at the orifice.

I have before observed, that I required my patients, in these cases, to lye upon their backs, and this, because, if they set up straight, the uterus would overset, and render the obstacle, if not invincible, at least, much more hard to remove.

However, both to ease my patients, and to prevent the child's ingaging itself too far in the pelvis, I get them, according to the circumstances, to keep still lain down, but to turn sometimes to one side, sometimes to the other, without ceasing my attentions, without discontinuing to rectify the turn of the internal orifice from over the summit of the child's head, and to uphold the said orifice, if it should tend to turn backwards, to depress it downward, by a gentle pressure, if it is inclined to rise towards the os pubis. This operation, this support, this depression, ought always to be managed with as much tenderness as skill, and there cannot be too much of both.

Certain it is, that the bad situation of the uterus often occasions a severe and difficult labor. A midwife therefore, from the very first of the labor-pains, cannot bestow too much attention to the giving such preventive or actual aid as I have proposed. Nothing, on these occasions, is more dangerous than delay. The pretious moments of operation must not be lost, least the child, coming to ingage itself, should throw us into an imbarrassment yet greater than the first.

In the beginning of the labor, it is no very great matter, to know exactly, what part the child presents to the orifice of an oblique uterus. It is enough to know, that it is not the head, in order to determine you, in due time, to the footling-extraction. What I mean is, that as soon as a good position shall have been procured to the orifice of the uterus; if it is any other part but the head that presents itself at that orifice, and that it is sufficiently dilated for the hand to get by gentle degrees introduced, dilated, in short, to about the diameter of a crown-piece, then, if the membranes do not break of themselves, the midwife should pierce them, and search for the feet of the child, to bring it away. But if the head it is that presents at the orifice, there is no need of any hurry: it is even better to wait till the membranes burst of themselves, unless they should be come out of the vagina, in which case they are to be opened, in order to terminate the delivery, not with scissors, but with the fingers alone.

The reader will here please to observe, that in these cases of obliquity, almost every thing depends, as to the prognostication, and prevention of difficulties, as well as to the relief in actual labor, on the exploration of the touch, and consequently the manual function. The last is especially and palpably indispensable. What can supply the place of it? not surely those forcing medicines, which some ignorant men-practitioners obtrude on the unhappy patient, and which only serve to exasperate the pains in vain, and certainly not to accelerate that parturition, which is retarded by the purely local indisposition of the womb. An obstacle which a skillful, tender, experienced hand cannot but be the fittest to remove.

In this case however it is, that Monsieur l'Accoucheur oftenest looks extremely silly and disconcerted. Though the throws redouble, the child is never the nearer coming out. On the contrary, till its passage is franked by the reduction of the uterus, it bears in vain upon any part, but that aperture, through which alone lies its issue: and, in fact, the harder it bears, the more it obstructs its own deliverance, and damages its mother. Monsieur l'Accoucheur stands by, does nothing, and can do nothing, or worse than nothing, if he should pretend to it: if he had the head, he has not the hand to give the patient any efficacious aid. Then it is, that where thus uncapable by Nature, for the manual function, the men-practitioners abuse that excellent, that divine, but here mistimed and misplaced maxim, of leaving things to Nature, of trusting to Nature. The power of Nature is just then, all of a sudden, acknowledged to be self-sufficient, when she really wants human help to redress her wrong. She is then at her greatest need, left to shift for herself. The fruitless pangs increase. Monsieur l'Accoucheur stands by an idle spectator, or perhaps goes about his business. In the mean time both mother and child, exhausted by fruitless efforts, for perhaps four, five, or six days, perish for want of the proper and only relief. Thus the ignorant operators abstain from interfering, when interfering, if they were fit for it, might be of service, only because they cannot so well in this case employ their iron or steel instruments: and as to their hands, they would most probably indeed make sad bungling work of it. Their action, in short, is, if that can be imagined, yet worse than their inaction.

Some of them, in this case, content themselves with saying, that the orifice is as yet too distant, and that nothing is urgent. They go away then, and leave the patient in the hope of some favorable change which is never to happen, They return, and find a strange disorder in the state of things, the child is too far engaged: it is too late to retrieve the damage, as they imagine, and I readily believe, when they have lapsed the due time of operation, of which not only probable they knew nothing, but, if they had known what to do, would have done it very ill. Then the vast knowledge and learning of these disconcerted instrumentarians can furnish them no better expedient, than that of murdering the child (as they pretend) to save the mother, though it is not always that the mother does not follow the fate of her poor infant.

I know, by my own experience, that often to make a happy end of such deliveries, requires an extreme attention and indefatigable pains. But practitioners should resolve, either to go through with the undertaking as it should be, or not begin it, in such cases, especially where the lives of mother and child depend upon their doing their duty, as they will answer the contrary to God, to man, and to themselves.

These cases are but too frequent in England. I have myself met with several of them, and sometimes even in persons extremely well made, in which I have been obliged to perform this manual aid, for many hours together, ay, even for half-a-day and more by the clock; all my motions keeping time with those of Nature narrowly watched, so as to rectify and adjust the orifice and the uterus; constantly reducing any detortion, and keeping things in their due direction. without tiring, or without losing patience.

Here I ask of my reader, is such work as this, naturally speaking, the work of a man, as Daventer would persuade us?

If the Monsieur l'Accoucheur is an ignorant, or rather not a very intelligent one indeed, the mother, or the child, or perhaps both, will probably be his victims.

But you say, if he is intelligent one all will be safe. No; he may perhaps know what to do, but will he have the woman's faculty of acquitting himself of his duty? all the theory in the universe will not do here without the practical part; and will the hands of a man in that respect ever equal the suppleness, the dexterity, the tenderness of a woman's? once more, is a man made for such work?

I say nothing here of the patience so remarkable in the true midwife on such trying occasions. I will grant, that Monsieur l'Accoucheur may, in the view of forty, fifty, or a hundred guineas perhaps, have enough of it not to slacken an attendance on his part, so dangerous, so insignificant, and often so pernicious; that it would be much better to pay him for his absence: I grant then, that he may employ his divine hippocratic fingers in such handy-work for so many hours together, without stepping into the next room for refreshment; or, in short, without hazarding the lives of the mother and child, by a remission of actual attention and manual assistance. But granting all this, can any one, who has a respect for truth, a respect for his own knowledge and sense of things, a respect, in short, for two such precious lives, as those of mother and child, not, I may say, intuitively, perceive and feel, the impropriety and danger of the practice, in such cases, being committed to a man preferably to a woman?

But would a woman especially, who loves herself, who loves the child in her womb, and who is capable of thinking at all, sacrifice herself and child to so palpable an imposition, as that of the pretended superiority of the men to the women in this point? She cannot even, well, without repugnance, submit, nor but for the indispensable necessity probably would submit to receive such service even from one of her own sex, whose tender, soothing, congenial softness, must make it more easy and supportable. But what can she expect from a man's clumsy, aukward, unnatural, disgustful operation, but increase of danger, or of pain, perhaps of both; while she and her child may not improbably be the victims of the rudiments in the art of a man by Nature condemned for ever to be a novice only, and who, for possibly a great hire to assist her, earns it only, as I have before observed, by excluding that due relief he is himself not capable of giving her; earns it by the not preventing enough her pains, and even by increasing her torments; till at length, not unfrequently, some infernal instrument is produced, like the dagger, in the fifth act of a tragedy, and forms the catastrophe of mother, or of child, or of both?

Of the **EXTRACTION** of the head of the **FOETUS**, severed from the **BODY**, and which shall have remained in the **UTERUS**.

I agree with our modern writers, that there can hardly exist a more vexatious accident, than that of the head's remaining in the uterus, after the extraction of the body. There are many causes of this effect. The death of the child for some time past, so that the waters may have had time to relax, to macerate the fibres, and thereby to render them incapable of resisting any efforts; there will result from thence a great difficulty of procuring the total issue of the dead fœtus, without dismembering it.

Some mis-conformation of parts in the mother may also contribute to it, or the obliquity of the uterus, where the child is brought away by the feet.

Independently of all these causes, this accident is almost always the effect of unskilfulness; it is, in truth, so rare, that it will scarce ever happen, where the delivery is conducted by an accurate and able practitioner of the art. If we have some examples, that even under skilful hands this case has come into existence, a thorough examination of it would shew, that it was only owing to the cruel necessity the practitioner may have been under, of being aided by persons not duly qualified to afford the least effectual help, or to conceive what they were directed to do.

But, however that may be, the damage is not absolutely without remedy. The great point is; without loss of time, to introduce the hand into the uterus, which does not proceed in its contraction, but gradually and leisurely enough, to give leave for the needful evacuation. It is true, that this operation requires a very nice skilful hand; with which, where it is found, surely no instrument, nor other invention, can come into competition.

This accident has appeared to occasion such severe labors, that many practitioners, and Peu, among others, (page 308) have advised abandoning the expulsion to Nature, rather than to fatigue the patient by fruitless and torturous attempts, to the success of which such obstacles presented themselves, as they looked upon to be unsurmountable.

Mauriceau (Aphor. 240) is of the same opinion, which he thus expresses. "When the head of the fœtus shall have remained in the uterus, which is no longer open enough to give it passage forth, it is better to commit the expulsion to Nature, than to attempt the extraction with too much violence."

These practitioners ground their opinion on that Nature, always wise and intent on self-preservation, taking more care to expel a superfluity, than even to attract the needful, often discharges herself, and that without violence, if she is but ever so little assisted, of all extraneous bodies, or other things retained in us against her intention.

Messieurs de la Motte, Peu, and Viardel adduce examples of Nature's doing spontaneously, what some of our later moderns are for absolutely doing themselves by means of those curious instruments, in which they make such a parade of the rare inventiveness of their genius, particularly in the extraction of a head remaining detached in the uterus, on its contracting some hours after the unskilful operation of some deficient practitioners. In such cases, I say, those gentlemen furnish instances of Nature's expelling the superfluous and extraneous incumbrance, with only the help of some glysters, and other remedies administered to the patient.

Now though no one can be more intimately convicted than I am, that Nature, acting for ever upon surer principles than Art, possesses resources which she often displays in the most desperate exigencies; I own, that in this case I am not for totally relying upon her beneficence[32]. Here is a wrong to redress, not owing to her, but to deficient practice; and this wrong can hardly be repaired by her alone, unless something of a better practice contributes to relieve her. That practice is not, however, the less recommendable for being plain and obvious. The most gentle, the most guarded, but withal the most efficacious means must be tried, little by little, to insinuate the fingers and hand into the uterus, how closely contracted soever it may be; for yield it will; and then seize the head by the mouth, the occipital cavity, or whatever other part affords the least slippery hold, without waiting whole hours, as do certain ignorant or negligent practitioners with respect to the after-birth, who give time to the uterus to enter into too strong contraction.

Some authors, and other persons of much that depth of practical merit, having learned solely by the experience of delaying to bring away the after-birth, that, to abandon thus the head of a child remaining in the uterus, was,

---

[32] It is but fair to observe, that M. De la Motte, (Obs. 248) instances, from Peu, two patients perished by the midwife's trusting to the pure actings of Nature in this very case.

at the same time, to expose the mother to the highest danger, judged it expedient to have recourse to auxiliary methods. They have therefore employed and directed for this purpose such edge-tools, as instruments and crotchets of different figures, some to incide and separate the bones of the skull; others to bring them away piece-meal, or all together, according as they should find the operation the easiest.

[33]Dyonis and Mariceau are of opinion, that the crotchet should be thrust into the most convenient place of the head, such as the mouth, one of the orbits of the eye, or the occipital cavity; after which, you are to endeavour to bring away the head by redoubled efforts. But if the crotchet slips, as the head is of a round figure, and may turn like a ball, they direct you to thrust the crotchet into the hole of the ear, then giving some one the handle to hold, you are to strike another crotchet of the same figure in the other ear, and so pulling with both crotchets at once, extract the head, that is to say, if possible.

Ay, that, "*if possible*," is well added; for with infinite submission to those very *learned* gentlemen, nothing appears to me more impracticable; and, I fancy, if they had ever made the experiment, they would have found it so. What a blind operation, with such instruments, and in such a place!

Guillemeau (Treat. of Mid. Book II. chap. 17.) remarks, that, in such case, you should take the time that the woman as a labor-pain to accomplish the extraction by this method, that is to say, to snatch that moment to extract the head, when you BELIEVE you have got fast hold of it.

But if the woman is too badly conformed, Dyonis (Book II. page 287) advises the use of the edged crotchets to cut the head to pieces, and bring away, by parts, what you could not do whole.

Mauriceau (Book II. page 287) would have it so, that this sort of crooked knife should have a long handle; and says, that Ambrose Paræus and Guillemeau are for a short one to it. Doctors will disagree. They all however give their respective reasons, and it is indeed hard to say which does not give the worst.

Mr. De la Motte, in the like circumstances, made use of a bistory, or incision-knife inserted in a sheath, open at both ends; of which he gives the following account. (Observ. 259)

---

[33] Dyonis in his Treatise, book III. ch. 12. Mauriceau, book II, chap. 14.

"I introduced, said he, into the uterus, my left hand, over which I fixed the head; and with my right, I slipped in a sheath open at both ends, in which was an incision-knife, that I applied to this head, and made an opening in it capable of admitting my fingers. I widened it afterwards, as much as I thought proper, and scooped out a part of the brain; after which, I got hold sufficient to bring away the head, of which the volume was considerably diminished."

Ambrose Paræus (Book of Gener. chap. 33.) tells us he had, to his great regret, a case of this sort fall to his share, the head of a fœtus remaining in the uterus. To extricate himself from which, he proposes much the same methods I have described after Dyonis and Mauriceau; and advises, in the same case, that if they do not succeed, recourse should be had to an instrument, called *pied de griffon*, (Griffin's claw) which he says he took from the French surgery of d'Alechamp. He gives two forms of one, one of two branches, another of four. These instruments, both the one and the other, are made on the principle of the *Speculum Matricis*[34], of which the use is at once, so detestably cruel, and so perfectly unavailing. The Griffin's claw however differs from the *speculum matricis*, in that the latter has its branches elbowing in an angle, and that the former has its branches streight a-top and at bottom, and arched in the middle, and furnished with roughnesses to seize and keep hold of the head.

Those who will take the trouble to see the delineation of these instruments, in these authors, will, at the very first glance of the eye, be convinced of their unserviceableness. So would they be of that of another instrument of the like nature, invented some years ago, and attributed to a surgeon of Rouen, which is composed of two crotchets, of which the blades are arched, and their extremities claw-footed.

The horror which these means of extraction naturally inspire, the damage and inconveniences inseparable from them, notwithstanding all the

---

[34] This instrument was once as much in vogue, as can be supposed of a time, when instruments were not so common as they are now. But how much torture in vain must it have given before it was discovered, that "so far from answering the *supposed* intention of it, namely, to extend the bones of the Pelvis; it can serve no other purpose than that of *bruising* or *inflaming* the parts of the woman." SMELLIE, p. 296.

Possibly the more modern instruments, which have supplanted this now exploded one, under the notion of improvement, will, in time be found to be liable to as just objection. But in the mean while what lives must be lost, what tortures endured, in the experiment! How many will have been the victims, women and children!

improvements pretended to have been made, have engaged several authors to imagine other less dangerous expedients. But before I mention them, I cannot well avoid taking notice of a suggestion of *Celsus*, if but to warn those whom it may concern, not to be too much carried away by the authority of a great *name*.

In such a case the method Celsus recommends, is, for one of the robustest men that may be got, to press strongly upon the belly of the patient, with his heavy hands, inclining them downwards, so that such a pressure may force out the head that shall have remained in the uterus. Is not this a right *learned*, and especially a very tender expedient?

Mauriceau and Amand giving a loose to their genius have proposed less perilous methods.

The first tells us, that it came into his head, in this case, that a fillet of soft linnen might be made, in form of a sling, to be slipped over the head, and so bring it away.

Amand has imagined a silk caul, of net work, to wrap the head in. This caul is to be pursed up by means of a string, that gathers four ribbons fastened to four opposite points of the circumference, or opening of this kind of purse, by which the head so wrapped up is to be extracted.

Mr. Walgrave professor at Copenhagen has improved on the first scheme of a fillet, by stitching together the two extremities of a fillet of linnen of about two yards long and four or five inches wide, in which he makes three slits lengthways, to seize the head more firmly, and hinder the fillet from slipping off the rounder parts of it. The figure of it may be seen in a Latin work intitled, *Dissertation upon the separated head of a child, and the different ways of extracting it from the mother's womb.* By Mr. John Voigt, at Gieffen, 1749.

Monsieur Gregoire, man-midwife at Paris, has disputed with Monsieur Amand the glory of this invention of the caul.

But if a reader will deign to consult his own reflexion, upon even these last, less however injurious means than those of iron and steel instruments, he will probably conclude, that if it is possible to come at the head, so as to fix, for example, a caul over it, the same liberty of access will serve to do all that can be necessary to secure a sufficient hold and purchase for the naked hand to bring it away, without such aids, as must necessarily suppose a free play of the hand in the uterus. I own this requires great shreudness of discernment by the touch, great expertness, great slight of hand and neat conveyance, but these are all points of excellence which midwives should be exhorted, encouraged, and even obliged to acquire: for acquire them they may; which is more than the men, generally speaking, ever can, and are therefore supplementally obliged to have recourse to such substitutes to hands, as those horrid instruments or silly inventions of theirs, with which, even at the best, they can never do so well as the women, who understand their business, can do without them.

Let it also be here remembered, what I observed at the beginning of this section, that this case of a separated head, I might almost say, never, no never comes into existence but through some previous neglect, error or failure of practice: so that surely the preventing it must be rather, preferable to the necessity of remedying it, either with crotchets, fillets, or even with but the hand alone; the trusting to any of which may make practitioners so often remiss, where remissness can hardly ever be but of bad consequence, where no fault, in short, can be other than a great one, and for which, the innocent patient it is that must most commonly be the sufferer, both in her own person, and in that of her child.

OF THAT LABOR IN WHICH THE HEAD OF THE FŒTUS REMAINS HITCHED IN THE PASSAGE, THE BODY BEING ENTIRELY COME OUT OF THE UTERUS.

It is here to be observed that though the body may be intirely free of the uterus, some of the causes deduced in the precedent section, may produce impediments or obstacles to the issue of the head. The head never detaches itself from the body but in that labor where the feet of the child come out first, and are too forcibly hauled by rash or unskilful hands, by such in short as do not know how to disingage or remove the let or obstacle to the issue of the head, with one hand, while with the other they properly support the body of the child. As it is then greatly to be wished that this accident might never happen, I shall, to the means I have already indicated for preventing or remedying it, add others coincidently with the design of this section, to prove the inutility of instruments in the case of the title prefixed to it. I shall then quote the practical tenets of the best authors upon this point, together with reflexions, which my own experience and practice have suggested to me.

162

Mauriceau explains this case tolerably justly, where he treats of the footling-extraction.

"Care (says he) should be taken that the child should have its face and belly directly downwards; to prevent, on their being turned upwards, the head of it being, towards the chin, stopped by the os pubis. If therefore it should not be so turned, it must be put into that posture. This will easily be done if, as soon as you begin drawing the child out by the feet, you incline and turn it little by little, in proportion as your extraction of it proceeds, till its heels bear in a direct line with the belly of the mother,"

[Here I must beg leave to interrupt Mr. Mauriceau, to observe, that it is not enough to have hold of the child's feet to begin turning it: but the breech must have come out: then, if it is not well turned, by placing one hand on the belly, and the other on the breech of the child, there will be time enough easily to turn it immediately and naturally, neither with too much precipitation, nor yet too leisurely, not little by little, or by slow degrees. This last precaution being of no use but to flag an operation, in which a delay may be fatal to the child, without any service to the mother, it only keeping her the longer in pain.]

"There are (he goes on) however children with so large a head, that it remains stopped in the passage after the body is intirely got out, notwithstanding all the precautions that can be used to avoid it. In this case, you must not stand amusing yourself with so much as attempting to bring the child away by the shoulders, for sometimes you will sooner part the body from the neck, than get the child out by this means. But while some other person shall pull it by the two feet or beneath the knees," *[here Monsieur Mauriceau is much out: great care should be taken not to have it pulled by any one, but purely to give the body of the child to be supported by some discret person, while the delivery proceeds as the author goes on to describe]* the operator will disingage little by little the head from between the bones of the passage, which he may do by sliding softly one or two fingers of his left hand into the mouth of the child, to disingage the chin in the first place, and with his right hand, he will embrace the back of the child's neck, above the shoulders, to draw it afterwards, with the help of one of the fingers of his left hand, employed, as I have just observed, in disingaging the chin. For it is this part which the most contributes to detain the head in the passage, whence it cannot be drawn out before the chin shall have been intirely disingaged. Observe also, that this is to be done with all possible dispatch for fear the child should be suffocated, as would indubitably happen, were he to remain any time thus held and stopped: because the umbilical chord, which will have come out, being turned cold, and strongly compressed by the body or by the head of the child, remaining too long in the passage, the child cannot then be kept alive by means of the mother's blood, whose motion is stopped in that chord, as well by its cooling which coagulates it, as by the compression which hinders it from circulating, for want of which it is a necessity for the child to breathe, which he cannot do till his head shall be intirely out of the uterus: therefore when once you have begun the extraction of the child, you must try to procure the total issue of it as quick as possible."

Monsieur Levret, who has wrote for no end on earth but to recommend his *tire-tête*, seizes the occasion of the foregoing passage extracted from Mauriceau to tell us, page 51, of the first part of his work.

"Mauriceau acknowledges here, that there are children who have the head so large, as for it to remain stopped in the passage, after the body shall have been wholly got out, notwithstanding all the precautions that can be taken to avoid it."

From whence this zealous instrumentarian draws the following conclusion. "Here (says he) is one of those cases, in which my *instrument* may be of great service."

This conclusion however does not to me at all appear a just one.

First, because Mauriceau, after those lines of his, just above quoted by Levret, adds immediately the method of practice pursuable in this case, to give a good account of it without the help of instruments.

Secondly, because we are not at all to be concluded by what any author says, any farther than the truth of things bears him out. Mauriceau[35] might

---

[35] Even this very Mauriceau allowed, by his brother practitioner M. De la Motte, to have been an excellent man-midwife, is however very justly animadverted upon by him for his weakness in giving into such nonsense, as prescribing histeric medicines by way of hastening the delivery. His capital receipt was the juice of a Sevile orange in an infusion of Sena. Let any one imagine, what an effect such a laxative potion must have on a woman, commonly rather wanting to have her strength recruited by proper restoratives, than diminished by purges, on so senseless a view. But how many other instances might be brought of these same most learned men-midwives, making almost a pitiful a figure in the character of physicians, as they must for ever do in that of manual practitioners of our art! Even the works of Daventer, who

164

have explained himself better: he might have said, that, in this case, the child should be pushed back a little into the uterus, to have the freer play for its being more easily disingaged: he might have advised, as I have before observed, rather a safer method of proceeding than what he has done. Mr. Levret himself allows this p. 56. Then, still with a view of recommend his forceps, his *tire-tête*, as being absolutely necessary, he continues thus (p. 58.)

"Though every thing should apparently have been done that is above set forth, still we are not always so happy as to accomplish the delivery. It sometimes happens, that we cannot get the head of the child out of the uterus. There are of this two examples in the treatise of M. De la Motte, of which I do not think it here out of place to furnish an extract.

"Mr. De la Motte, in his 253d. Observation, (goes on M. Levret) relates, that in a case in which he was obliged to turn the child, in order the better to finish the delivery, he turned it very easily; that having brought it out as far as to the thighs...it being alive, he gave its body a half turn, so as to put its face downwards which it had upwards, and that then he continued drawing out the child as far as to the shoulders and neck.

After that (says M. De la Motte) I gave it some gentle shakes, and even pulled it pretty hard, and had several tugs at it, to make an end of a delivery I had so happily begun; but all was in vain. This obliged me, according to my usual method, to put my finger into its mouth. I was mistaken, for what I took to be the mouth, I found to be the nape of the neck, and that the neck, not having followed the motion of the body, was twisted round, and consequently the face still remained turned upwards, so that the chin it was that, being hitched at the os pubis, was the obstacle to have been conquered to terminate the delivery."

MR. Levret here observes, there being a great probability that, when la Motte turned the body of the child, he was pulling it towards him, and that the mother was in a labor-throw: for it is well known, that then the uterus contracts itself in all directions round the body it contains: she was then

---

has such glimpses of true theory, prove him not uninfected with a spice of quackery. This is generally speaking so true of the men-dabblers in practical midwifery, that one would imagine the extension of that meanness of theirs, in putting their nose into such a function, even to their collateral profession, whatever it be, of physician, surgeon, chemist or apothecary, was the revenge of Nature, for the outrages of their pretended art upon her.

compressing exactly the head of the child, which must render it immovable, while he was turning the body. These two co-incidences must have contributed to twist the neck of the child, consequently to make it lose its life. And to clench the misfortune, he gave its little body to be held by the husband of the mother, while he was pushing back the head with one hand, and with the other disengaging the chin. He told the husband at the same time to pull softly; "but he hauled with such violence, in the hope of easing his wife, that he fell with a jerk six foot off the bed, with the body of the child, of which the head had remained in the uterus."

Let us proceed to the second example. This is the fact. M. De la Motte tells us, that he was called to assist a poor woman in labor, in which she had lingering for two days, that this patient was a very little woman, and of about forty five years of age; the arm of a very small child had come out the day before.

"I slipped (said he) my hand along this little arm, to go in quest of the feet, which I presently found, and after having closed them together, I brought them away out of the uterus. The body followed till it came to the neck. The patient being on the edge of the bed, which was very high from the ground, and where there was not room enough left to support the child in proportion as I drew it out, I was obliged to give it a woman to hold, while I proceeded gently to disingage the head which was stopped in the passage. This was no wonder, considering the streightness of it, being correspondent to the littleness of her size; considering withal the advanced age of the patient, the length of time since the discharge of the waters, during which the uterus being irritated by the lingeringness of the labor, the presence of the arm in the passage had caused an inflammation, consequently some induration, all these joined to the time that the fœtus had been dead, which as before observed was a very small creature, were reasons more than sufficient to manage very tenderly with the child, so as to bring it away whole. This (says M. De la Motte) induced me to introduce my hand flat towards the *frænum laborium*, and to put my middle finger into the child's mouth, while my other hand was over its neck. My measures being thus taken, I desired the midwife, while I should disingage the parts, to pull softly, for fear of an accident. But she nevertheless, senselessly and foolishly, gave it much such a pull, as the woman's husband I have before mentioned. This indeed forced out the body of the child, but severed from the head, which remained in the uterus."

Here it may be observed that Monsieur Levret, by this preamble, on the one hand prepares us for the necessity of his instrument, by a constant supposition of cases, in which, notwithstanding all the precautions that may be taken, it happens sometimes (as he says) "that it is not possible to terminate happily the delivery, nor get the child's head out of the uterus;" to support which opinion he produces the two examples from De la Motte, which I have just before quoted.

On the other hand, he owns, as it were, *en passant*, that there are means, which he even explains of accomplishing successfully the deliveries, in such labors, by solely the operation of the hands, avoiding the faults committed by M. De la Motte, after which, as if those faults were any proof in favor of his instrument, he concludes, that, "if through any cause whatever, this case was not to be got over, the child should be given to some one to be held, with the precautions before set forth, and that then the operator was to proceed with his instruments."

In the first example we see that De la Motte was guilty of three grievous errors. The first, in taking the nape of the neck for the mouth: the second, in having taken the time of the mother's throw, in which the uterus must have contracted round the neck in all directions, to turn the body of the child, which contributed to twist its neck: thirdly, in having given the body of the child to the husband to hold, with direction to pull it, even tho' he cautioned him to do it gently. He ought rather not to have trusted him with the body at all, or have absolutely forbid him to make the least motion, his part being only to support it.

In the second example, De la Motte committed no more than the last fault, in trusting a midwife, of whom he might not know all the stupidity: but this was sufficient to produce that accident; an accident which it will not even be hard to avoid, with due management, or hands skilfully conducted.

With Mons. Levret's leave (whom I ought to honor, since it is from him I have chiefly taken what he has said against all instruments but his own) I shall then say, that it is against the laws of candor, or of common sense, to seek, from the faults which may be committed in the manual practice, either through ignorance, inadvertence, or want of circumspection, to infer the necessity of instruments.

167

The point here under discussion turns intirely upon a child extracted by the feet. Now it is extremely rare, that in this case, the head does not follow the body. But if, in exception to this general rule, the head should be stopped in the passage, upon proceeding to disengage it, with all the proper measures and precautions which I have added to those above specified from Mauriceau, the sole aid of the hands will be full sufficient to accomplish the total delivery. But if they were to be ill managed, the risk would be evidently great of detaching the body from the head; and this would change the case from that of the head stuck in the passage, to the one of the head separated from the body, of which I have treated in the preceding section. Without then multiplying cases without necessity, as the reader will easily see, that the first is but the consequence of a mis-treatment of the last, so that, by the same rule, the right management of the last case is a sure prevention of the first, I shall only observe, that it might be shewn, that capable, well-conducted hands are sufficient to guard against both dangers, and shewn, even by Mons. Levret's own confession, which he so inconsistently contradicts, in favor of his own instrument, without offering any thing like a reason for such a contradiction.

But if the damage in these cases resulting from an unskilful use of the hands should be urged against me: I answer, in the first place, that I am not arguing for any thing but what is to be effectuated by good practice: my point, is only to establish the superiority of skilful hands to the use of instruments: and in these cases, I aver, that even the damages done by the mis-practice of defective hands, may be better repaired by sufficient ones, than by a recourse to instruments. How often too are instruments used by such men-operators, as are to the full as unfit to manage such instruments, bad as they are, as some women may be to use their hands! But if I could give no better reason for the rejection of instruments, than the abuse of them, even by the numbers of ignorant superficial men-practitioners that employ them, I should not expect to be heard; and yet the great argument against midwives is the ignorance of a few of them: though that ignorance of theirs could never produce such a multiplicity of horrors, of murders, injuries, tortures of mothers, such mutilations and massacres of children, as the deep learning of the instrumentarians!

My plea then is much more fair. The reader will be pleased to consider, and decide upon his own reflexions, whether, it is not at least probable, from what has been shewn in the cases of the obliquity of the uterus, of a head separate from the body of the fœtus, or even of that reputed most dangerous extremity, the head being hitched in the passage, when the whole body shall have come out, that every thing may be at least as hopefully attempted with the hands alone, as with those instruments, the use of which forms the sole reason for a recourse to men-practitioners; tho', well considered, nothing could be a stronger reason against such a recourse than their using them. But let us proceed to the next case;

WHEN THE HEAD OF THE FŒTUS PRESENTS ITSELF FOREMOST, BUT STICKS IN THE PASSAGE.

For this section it is, that I have reserved to treat incidentally and more at large of the objections to be made in general to all instruments, and in particular to the principal ones.

Among the severe labors, which give much trouble, and exact much patience from all parties, from the patient, the midwife, and all the assistance, this case may challenge a place. It is that, in which the head of the child having presented itself foremost, and having ingaged itself half way, or thereabouts, in the streight of the bones of the pelvis, and of the orifice of the uterus, the labor-pains remit, languish, and the progress of the labor becomes suspended. Whether there be any mis-conformation of the bones of the pelvis, or whether (as our practitioners are pleased to express it,) the head of the fœtus be too large for the passage, or whether, in short, both these causes concur to the formation of this obstacle, or exist in complication with other circumstances; it is, in this case, we may say the head is hitched, stuck or ingaged in the passage.

Mr. De la Motte, book the 3d. chapter the 20th, describes this state of the fœtus.

"When (says he) the head has struck into the streight of the passage which, at first, affords a great deal less room than were to be wished, for its letting it pass, the head ingages itself as much forward as possible, from the continual and violent pains the woman suffers, which act upon the child, whose head lengthens and flattens, in such a manner, to adjust and mould itself to the passage, that the hairy scalp becomes quite tumefied, so as to make the head look almost like a double head, which however remains stuck fast between the

169

bones, without being able to get out, and only ingages itself the more the more it advances...but growing larger as it advances, and the aperture which it obliged to force diminishing more and more, makes it so that the head remains at length so jammed in, that it cannot be drawn out without diminishing its volume, which (as this author says) cannot be executed without instruments: as I was obliged to do, to accomplish the following delivery."

Mr. De la Motte then proceeds to tell us, that he was called to lay the wife of a laborer, the head of whose child was hitched in the passage. After having well examined the state of the mother and child, and ascertained as much as it is possible to ascertain the death of the latter—"I determined, (says he) to finish the delivery, which I did by opening the head of the child with my incision-knife, and scooped out therewith part of the brain. After which, I made use of my hand, with which I got hold of the inside of the skull, and in an instant drew the child out, who appeared to have been dead a long time."

It is not here that, in answer to M. De la Motte, I shall stop to propose a more gentle and more natural method of giving a good account of this case of a hitched head, than the cruel and dangerous expedients suggested by the instrumentarians: I reserve the submission to better judgment of my own ideas of practice, in this point, till after I shall have quoted the notions of more authors.

Daventer, p. 343, of his observations, supposes to us the case of a head stuck in the passage, when the difficulty of the labor shall have been increased, as well by the ignorance, as by the negligence practitioner, male or female, that may not have given the proper aid in due time, or not have foreseen the danger; he moreover supposes a complication of obliquity, caused by the mis-conformation of the bones in the patient. If this embarrassment then should not have been foreseen or guarded against, he advises the opening of the head of the child.

"There is, for this no occasion (says he) for any instruments of a particular make; a common knife guarded as far as the point, a pair of scissors, a pointed spatula do the business. The opening they make may be dilated with the fingers, and the brain taken out; after which, you seize the head with your hand, or with a linnen cloth, and try, in this manner, to bring away the body. When I say you may draw the head out with a linnen cloth, I mean a broad strip or fillet cut lengthways of the cloth, and hemmed in the borders,

170

or any piece of linnen that is fine and strong, to be passed round the back of the head, and bringing in under the chin, you twist the fillet, and draw out the child."—He then adds, that he much esteems this method; that those, whose hands are *small* enough to pass this linnen round the back of the head, without opening it, are not obliged to open it, and have therein a great advantage over others.

This last method proposed by Daventer ought doubtless to be preferably pursued, as being the less cruel. But, in the first place, it is utterly impracticable. A head represented to be hitched or jammed, does not leave the least hands that can be imagined room or liberty to pass a fillet round the back of the head, in order to bring it under the chin. But were it even practicable, it would be useless, and dangerous: useless, in that the hands alone, so introduced, might of themselves, little by little, disingage this head; dangerous, for that this fillet might most likely produce the effect that fillets commonly do, strangle the child.

Mauriceau, to conquer this obstacle of the head so stuck, proposes several kinds of crotchets, to apply various ways, to the head of the child, after having scooped out the brain, by means of an opening made in the scull. He gives us several examples in his observations, but as they are absolutely fit for nothing but to inspire horror, I shall refrain from specifying them. Dyonis is of the same opinion with Mauriceau.

Those who will give themselves the trouble to peruse the authors who have preceded thus, will find, that their method differs very little from that of la Motte and Mauriceau, which most assuredly kills the child if it is not dead: and the ascertainment of the death of a child stuck in the passage is so difficult, that the ablest practitioners cannot answer for not being mistaken in it. The reader will please to apply here what I set forth, p. 139, and following, to which I beg leave to refer.

Mauriceau, at length, imagined, that he had out-done all others, in his invention of an instrument he calls a *tire-tête*. He specifies it in his 26th observation. But it is as dangerous as the crotchets, since, in order to use it, you must begin by opening the skull with an incision-knife, or with a sort of steel spike, double-edged, which he invented on purpose for the use of piercing the child's scull at the *fontanelle*, to admit a little round plate of steel of another instrument.

Monsieur Soumain, and other celebrated practitioners, have acknowledged the insufficiency of this instrument of Mauriceau; but were it good for any thing; as to drawing out the head so stuck, it would for ever be fatal to those poor unfortunates, since it could not fail of killing them if they were still alive.

After this we have the tire-tête of Mr. Fried, but it is as murderous as that of Mauriceau, nor answers the intentions which its author had proposed to himself. He has therefore himself had the candor to condemn it, as may be seen p. 154. in a treatise of midwifery, published in 1746, by the care of Mr. Boëhmer, who has added two dissertations to the treatise on this art by Dr. Manningham.

Mr. Menard, in his preface, p. 24, gives the figure of an instrument, of which the idea seems to have been taken from a twibill, with a ducks beak. Mr. Menard has endeavoured at perfecting it, by having it made angular, shortened, and grooved. He has given it a figure of dented pinchers, with curve claws. He gives us also the figure of an instrument pointed and edged, made like the head of a spear, which he uses for opening the scull, and introducing the pinchers, by means of which he draws the child out by the head, as he keeps pinching the bones of the scull and teguments. By this it is easy to conceive, that this instrument has no advantage over that of Mauriceau, and has all its inconveniences.

Many other modern practitioners advise the use of one or two crotchets, be the child dead or alive, or of a tire-tête, made in form of strait blades, with spoon-bills, to introduce them one after another into the uterus; and after having placed them on each side of the child's head, and made them meet together, to try the extraction with them.

This last contrivance, as ingenious as it may appear, does not save the child's life, as all these authors would insinuate. For these instruments, wherever they are applied, must pierce to get a solid hold; without they could serve for nothing but to crush or lacerate the teguments; so that they should not be used where the child is a live one: and even when it's dead, the mother is not absolutely safe from the damage they may do, whatever precaution the operator may take, or whatever may be his dexterity of hand. If one of the blades should slip, which frequently happens, it will be difficult for him not to do the mother a mischief. For as to the child, it is very rare that the crotchet does not instantly destroy it.

Menard has again given us another figure of an instrument, to appearance less dangerous; but the make of it sufficiently denotes its want of power in the operation, which is also confirmed by the testimony of the most celebrated practitioners.

It is now (1760) about forty years ago, that Palfin, a surgeon of Ghent in Flanders, and demonstrator of anatomy in the same town, went to Paris, and there presented to the academy of sciences an instrument for extracting, by the head, children stuck in the passage. Gilles le Doux, surgeon of the town of Ypres, put in his claim to the invention of this curious instrument, which has however been ever looked upon as insufficient, and to have too much bulge, to allow its introduction into a place already so difficult by its being blocked up with the body that requires the extraction. After at least a dozen of corrections of this pretended tire-tête or forceps of Palfin, Gilles le Doux himself corrected it, so did afterwards Messieurs Petit, Gregoire, Soumain, Dussé, and I do not know how many more.

In short, one may say, that never did any instrument undergo more alterations than this forceps has done. One of the greatest improvements, according to the opinion at the time here in England, which it received, was that given it by Dr. Chamberlain. Chapman, whose treatise on midwifery is esteemed, to give this tire-tête the greater lustre, tells us, that Dr. Chamberlain kept this instrument a long while a secret; and that the Dr's father, his two brothers, and himself, used it with good success. Mr. Boëhmer, public professor of physic and anatomy at Hall, in the Lower Saxony, in the College Royal of Frederic, and of the society of curious Naturalists, from whom I quote this, calls this instrument, I am here speaking of, the English tire-tête, or forceps.

All due honor be to the original author of this sublime invention of the forceps, whoever was the happy mortal! Happy, I say, according to Dr. Smellie, who calls it a *"fortunate contrivance"*[36]; though perhaps by fortunate, he rather means its having been so to himself. For hitherto, in all truth, I must own, that I do not find, even by the most exaggerated accounts of the learned men-midwives, that those poor instruments of God's making, the women fingers, would not much better, and much safer, do every thing that is

---

[36] Page 249, of his treatise of midwifery.

pretended to be done by that same boasted instrument, or that can be done by any other human means.

But let us suppose for an instant, what both my love and knowledge of the truth would hinder me from granting, that instruments are at some times, and in some sort necessary: in what case is it that they are necessary? this is what hitherto I do not know. And which instrument is it that a man-midwife must use? that is what I yet know less: nor do I believe there is any practitioner so presumptuously silly, as to admit any particular one, as the only one universally received and approved. It will perhaps be said, that according to the circumstances, each practitioner will, out of his bag of hard-ware, pick out that which will be fit for the occasion. But then, a waggon would not carry their whole armory, to calculate not only according to the various alterations made, if but in the forceps, by whim, desire of getting a name, or of encreasing practice, but according to the various exigencies and circumstances to which the form of the instrument ought to be peculiarly adjusted. And upon every occasion, there is not the time for inventing, directing, or making a new instrument. But if it is said, that for want of such exactness, the general make of an instrument must do, in *all* cases: that general make is not at least to be looked for in any of the kinds I have already quoted, by which such numbers of women and children must have been tortured or sacrificed, before they were exploded and given up, as good for nothing or insufficient, even by the men-practitioners themselves, who however substituted no others to them but what were rarely less exceptionable. They were only newer. Let us then now proceed to pass in a summary review the later and pretended improvements of this prodigious invention of the forceps, and candidly examine the validity of their claim over the women's hands.

Mr. Rathlaw, a famous surgeon of Holland, in his dissertation on the means, or secret of Roger Roonhuysen, which was transmitted to his heirs, for extracting (as was said) in a very little time, a child, whose head should be embarrassed in the neck of the uterus, says thus,

"To me it appeared impossible, to establish an instrument, whose use should be so certain, so general, so necessary, that one could not be a man-midwife without having a knowledge of it."

The same Mr. Rathlaw, in the same piece, exclaiming against the use of the crotchets has this remark.

"No one (says he) can be ignorant of it's being no longer the practice in France, or in England, to employ crotchets, or murderous tire-têtes (*would this were truth!*) in the deliveries, unless for a monstrous or hydrocephalous head, when the bulk of it is so enormous, that there is no possibility of getting it out whole, and especially if the child should be dead... In my time (adds this author) every eminent man-midwife had invented different means of extracting himself out of the plunge of such a case, and their reputation grew in proportion to their respective success. Yet, Hitherto, I do not know, that either at Paris or at London, they have got such a length, as to take any particular instrument under their protection. Nine years ago, (Mr. Rathlaw continues) I had made a forceps almost wholly of my own invention to extract the fœtus by the head, and it often succeeded well with me. It was, as to its make, a good deal resembling that which Butter describes in the Edinburgh-acts, volume III. art. 20. But mine (proceeds he) seem to possess better proportions, and is certainly of a more handy use, than those which have hitherto appeared."

Please to observe, that this forceps of Mr. Rathlaw is the same as Palfin's, or rather as that of Gilles le Doux, excepting only the semilunar hollow cuts in the claws, which Monsieur Dussé, a surgeon of Paris, had contrived in them. The author says, it had *often* succeeded well with him: he does not say *always*, and why? most probably because, when he did so *often* find it of service, that was; only whenever there was no sort of occasion for using it at all. Do not let it here be imagined, that I force an inference. I give my reason. Supposing that such an instrument was necessary to every practitioner, the case for his using it cannot but rarely occur. Now those rare cases where Rathlaw judged his forceps necessary, and in which it failed him, were in all likelihood the true tests of its merit: whereas those other cases, in which he *often* succeeded, may very well be taken for such as, with hands and patience, might have afforded a better account of them, than the silly superfluous quackery of employing a forceps, unless indeed his hands were too clumsy to attempt it. Otherwise the using instruments, where they sometimes do the work with so much more pain and danger, when the bare hands well conducted would do so much better, remind me naturally enough of what I have seen a pretty master do with a steel-instrument called a zig-zag or fruit-tongs, when, to display it, or out of wantonness, he has catched up fruit with it, that lay fully within the reach of his hand. In this piece of childishness there is however no mischief; whereas the man-midwife, for considerations of lucre, dallies with two lives to pluck at a fruit that is never, I repeat it, never, out of reach of the hand, where that steel-instrument of his, a forceps, can bring it away.

Mr. Rathlaw also tells us of another instrument, of which he gives us an account. He had got the secret from one Velsen, a physician at the Hague. This Velsen had it of Vanderswam, who had been a pupil of Roonhuysen, the inventor of this pretended nostrum, with which he always helped the women in labor, snug under the bedcloaths, the better to conceal his miraculous secret. He had long promised his pupil to discover it to him.

"In short (says Mr. Rathlaw) one day that Roonhuysen was returning from laying a woman, a burgomaster of Amsterdam came to speak with him: in the hurry Roonhuysen was to receive him, he did his nostrum-instrument in some apartment. His curious pupil (Vanderswam) who had for several years been watching such an occasion with great eagerness, found it, and took a draught of it. This instrument was in a case with two long steel crotchets, and a piece of whale-bone, in the shape of a pipe for smoking, only shorter, and at one of the ends of which was a piece of steel, of the shape of an acorn, and there was no other instrument in this case."

If Mr. Velsen is to be believed, it seems, on the one hand, that Roonhuysen made the whole science of midwifery consist in the knowledge and use of this his instrument, since it is there said, that Roonhuysen had promised this pupil of his to teach him the art of midwifery, but taught him nothing of it; and indeed it does not appear, that he had hidden any thing from Vanderswam but this wonderful instrument, with which he used, under the bed-cloaths, to smuggle the child through difficult passage[37].

On the other hand again, it may be judged, that this pretended marvellous instrument was not of effectual enough service to its inventor, unless in those cases where he might as well have done without them, since this very same Roonhuysen made use of crotchets, doubtless, when he found his instrument

---

[37] That is to say, if he touched the woman at all with it, and did not sometimes, at least, *make believe* that he delivered her with it though Nature alone should have done the work. Sure I am that that piece of quackery in him of pretending to hide the instrument, might justify such a suspicion, of a less guilt however than that of really applying an instrument insignificant to any purpose but that of torture in vain.

fail him. O women! women! thus it is that your pretious lives, and that of your children (to say nothing of the additional tortures you are put to, as if those of Nature's own ordering were not already enough) are trifled with, in practices being tried upon you with such instruments, for which you are besides to pay exorbitantly; and all for what? To encrease the practice of some quack, who raises into notice his worthless name, or perhaps swells some work of his, published by way of advertising himself, with the rare boast of having delivered you with an instrument, that has only, not murdered some of you, though it may sometimes perhaps have done you irreparable damage, and will have always occasioned you an unnecessary increase of pain and danger. Is it possible to inculcate this truth too often or too strongly to you?

"There are many people, (adds Mr. Rathlaw) who make a doubt whether this instrument is not the same as that with which the three Chamberlains, brothers, acquired in Ireland and other countries the reputation of being the most eminent men-midwives in the world. In those circumstances in which others employed crotchets, they could, by their manual operation, and with less labor, hasten the delivery of the women in less time, and without the least danger to mother and child."

I am not unwilling to believe that the three brothers, the Chamberlains, might pass for the most eminent men-midwives in the world, especially in Ireland, where before there never had, as I understand, been seen any practitioners of midwifery but women. As to other countries, these brothers might very easily surpass in skill those, who knew no gentler way of terminating a delivery than by the means of crotchets. Therefore it is that our author adds, that the Chamberlains only made use of the manual operation; he does not add of other instruments. It is a great pity however, that the surgeons of all countries have not yet got hold of, and adopted this marvellous secret of Roonhuysen's, which would extricate them so gloriously, in their attendance on such difficult labors. They would thereby greatly reduce their armory, from its complex state at present of variety of crotchets, tire-tête, forceps, spoons, blunt hooks, pinchers, fillets, lacs, scissors, incision-knives, and the rest of their tremendous apparatus.

According then to Mr. Rathlaw, the forceps of Roonheysen was the same as that of the Chamberlains. How he got the secret from them matters not. He only changed the figure of the blade-parts. In short, our author adds, that to him it seems probable, that this instrument has been brought to perfection by the continual experience of men-midwives, who have successively employed it. He pretends himself to have made some alterations in it for the better, but what they are he is not pleased to tells us.

The illustrious Janckius, a great practitioner, mentions another corrected forceps in his dissertation upon the forceps and pinchers, instruments invented by Bingius, a surgeon of Copenhagen, and of their use in difficult labors, printed at Leipsic, 1750, page 211. This forceps resembles mostly that which the celebrated Monsieur Gregoire, senior, first imagined upon the model of Palfin's tire-tête.

"Janckius, in the same dissertation, tells us, that it would be of service to have spoons or blades of the forceps of various curvatures, and of different lengths, for the shorter the arching, and more crooked the blades or spoons are, the more difficult and dangerous will the application be, according to Chapman and Boëhmer."

Thence this consequence seems derivable, that to obviate these difficulties and dangers, it would be requisite to have as many crooked spoons as there are particular cases, as well as to take measure of the heads that are stuck, which still would imply the introduction of the hand, and, of course, the uselessness of instruments.

Mr. Levret, in his notes, p. 377, makes us observe, that the branches of the forceps of Bingius, which are solid, being considerably more crooked than the windowed forceps, the expansion of their middle part must be too wide not to risque, in the extraction, the *tearing* the perinæum, which it is no such *indifferent* matter as not to be remarked.

This Janckius had, it seems, that bad habit of employing too *soon* the instrument of Bingius, which is extremely dangerous. This however, is not seldom the case, when Monsieur l'Accoucheur is in a hurry.

Boëhmer, in a dissertation on this subject, thus expresses himself, as to the instrument of Levret, and the forceps of Bingius.

"I shall only observe (says that learned physician) what Mr. Leveret has himself very justly remarked, that the application of the forceps is dangerous, unless the head should have already descended low enough into the pelvis for the orifice of the uterus to be effaced, and to make but one and the same cavity with the vagina. This counsel is essential for two reasons;

"First, for fear of hurting the orifice of the uterus which might easily happen without this precaution.

"Secondly, on account of the instrument itself, the blades of which could not embrace more than a part, and not the whole of the head, which remaining too high, they could not consequently compress it equally, nor extract it. It is for the same reasons (continues he) that I rather differ in opinion from the celebrated Janckius, who, as soon as the waters are discharged, and he perceives that the head does not pass, has instantly recourse to the instrument... Some time (says he) should be indulged to the action of Nature... There is often more success obtained by temporising, than by too early a recourse to instruments."

Little by little the truth will come out. Little by little, even the men-practitioners themselves, will be forced to allow, that the very least imperfect of the instruments are prejudicial and dangerous: though perhaps they will not speak out the whole truth, and confess that total uselessness, which would, in so great a measure, imply their own. But commonsense will inform whoever consults the light of it within himself, that these instruments are of a nature so heterogeneous, from the service expected from them, so impossible to be adapted to the infinitely tender texture of the organ of gestation, that the very best of them must occasion lacerations, especially by the opening of the branches, the strain of which bears upon the mother's body, and can never but hurt the child, in crushing it's head; as they make that to be done precipitately, about which Nature has, for taking her own longer time, no doubt a very good reason, if there was no more than that one of gradually dilating the passage; but there are probably many others.

Art should aim at imitating Nature: now Nature proceeds leisurely, instead of which the forceps goes too quick to work. The action of it depends on an artificial compression, which begins by moulding, or rather crushing the child's head, adaptingly to the figure of the pelvis, to facilitate its extraction; and though the divine providence has in its wisdom provided for the preservation of the human species, by means of what is called the durameter, and by the void of the sutures in the cranium of children, the manual compression of the instrument is either too strong or too weak. If too strong, the child is lost; the head being so compressed by the instrument, that the brain escapes through the occipital cavity: if it is too weak, so that the head has not been sufficiently compressed, nor it's bulk competently diminished, in attempting the extraction, not only the uterus can scarce escape the being wounded, but the perinæum and the bladder the being torn: and indeed in either case they hardly escape, the instruments occasioning various inflammations and contusions, of the worst consequence, both in the internal and external parts, besides the great danger of the blades flipping and violently hurting the mother, not to mention the painful divarications and shocking attitudes in order to the introduction.

The instrument used by Mr. Giffard, man-midwife, is supposed by Levret and others to be nothing more than the windowed forceps, of which the use had been long before known. But that appears as unsatisfactory as others. Mr. Freke too, it seems, furnished a new kind of corrected forceps, the chief merit pretended of which was, that the extremity of one of the blades was curved in form of a crotchet, and that this extremity might be *concealed* when not employed as a crotchet, and consequently helped to avoid the having a multiplicity of instruments, as this new-fangled one might, upon an occasion, serve either for crotchet or forceps.—What a prodigious strain of sublime invention is this of death and wounds in various shapes!

I find too that Chapman is blamed, for that, in his essay on the art of midwifery, he very frankly condemns all the tire-têtes he had seen employed till his time by all other practitioners, but he has not, it seems, given a description of the one he himself used, nor doubtless the method of using it, the one necessarily depending on the other. Nor where that author speaks of passing a ribbon over the head of a child, is he so good as to tell you how he managed to get it over.

I must not here omit some mention of the forceps, pretended to be improved by Dr. Smellie. Upon which, however, I shall spare the reader a tedious minute discussion of its form, and of its advantages and disadvantages, comparatively to other forceps calculated for the same use. Levret may to the curious furnish sufficient satisfaction on that head. He has examined it with great exactness and seeming candor, even though he prefers his own to it. Nothing can be plainer, than its being just as insignificant and foolish a gimcrack as any of the rest. But there is one particularly, of which Levret takes notice, that I cannot well omit mentioning. The Dr. has, it seems, whether to spare the women the shock of the gleam from a polished steel instrument, or, whether defend them from the injury of the metalline chill, which is not well to be cured by any warming at the fire, covered his instrument with leather spirally wound round it. Levret upon this concludes his remarks with the following one. "The ledges or roughness which the leather must, *besides increasing its bulk*, create by those its spiral circumvolutions, cannot but be such an obstacle to the introduction of the instrument, as to let it be serviceable only in those cases where (N.B.)—one may do *very well without* it. For it is well known, than in those cases where recourse to it is requisite, the most polished, the most smooth instrument often finds such great difficulties in its intromission, that nothing but a hand, *consummately* expert in the use of this instrument[38] can, without damage, remove the impediments."

Dr. Smellie has, however, himself salved one of Levret's objections to his instrument, as to any offensive smell or infection that might be contracted by the use of it. (Treatise of Mid. p. 291.) The "blades of the forceps ought to be *new covered* with stripes of *washed* leather, after they shall have been used, especially in delivering a woman suspected of having an *infectious* distemper." Certainly, certainly, not only the Doctor's nine hundred pupils, but all other practitioners, that use this famous instrument, will do well to observe this injunction. It is the very best thing they can do, next to never using it at all.

I come now to the boasted instrument of Levret; who is the last, at least that I know of, who has invented a new make of a tire-tête, or forceps corrected, over all that have appeared since Palfin. He gives us, in a book written on purpose to recommend it, a minute analysis of it, and an ingenious delineation in some pretty prints of it. The work is intitled, *Observations sur les causes et les accidents de plusieurs accouchemens laborieux.*

But to make use of the instrument or instruments which Levret recommends, requires not only a hand consummately dexterous and skilful in the art, but an infinite number of perplexing precautions, as may be seen, p. 106, and seq. of his observations.

I will not here undertake a circumstantial account, I shall content myself with mentioning some of them.

"There is here (says our author) a very important remark to be made, when you are for using this forceps. It is absolutely necessary that the orifice of the

---

[38] How few are there such? consequently how great the danger of such instruments, even if they were good for any thing, to be introduced into *common* practice?

uterus should be, as it were, totally effaced or crazed, that is to say, that the vagina and the uterus should, in a manner, no longer form other than one and the same cavity, from a sort of uninterrupted continuity, because, without that, there would be a danger of getting hold of the orifice of the uterus between the head of the child and the instrument, which would be extremely hurtful.

"I ought (continues he) to add, that great attention should be given to the attention of that orifice, for before it's intirely disappearing, it becomes sometimes so thin, and so exactly close fitted to the child's head, that, without a most scrupulous examination, one might commit a mistake."

Besides the measures, observations and remarks this practitioner urges in that place, which require infinite attentions, he adds to them the following ones.

"First, when you introduce the instrument you are never sure of being in the uterus, but, when, besides the precaution I have above recommended, you feel that the axis of the instrument, or the extremity of the branches, is in a kind of vacuum. This sign would I own be a very equivocal one, for a person that should use this forceps without having practised surgery[39]; but so it will not be for him, whose sense of the touch is habituated to the feeling of instruments of different sorts, as they enter into empty cavities of vessels or of hollow organs, or in short of any cavity.

"Secondly, when by drawing towards yourself the instrument, you are assured of the preceding sign, you will feel a small resistence to a certain degree.

"Thirdly, the blades of the instrument should suffer themselves to be opened out with some sort of ease, and what is opened out should not make resistence enough for the blades to return with any violence to the place whence the opening out began.

"Fourthly, the blades in the instrument should, as they open wider and wider, rather tend to augment the diameter of the void of the instrument than diminish it.

"Fifthly, these same blades should, in their expansion, go a little depth in the vagina.

"If the man-midwife, (says Levret) perceive, that *any* of these favorable signs should be *wanting*, he ought to *mistrust* the *success*, and to have recourse to his *sagacity* for the remedying it."

---

[39] As the practice of midwifery is, properly speaking, under no regulation, may not this be too often the case?

Thus far as to the handling this forceps of Levret's, to whom the defectiveness of the English and French forceps had inspired an idea of providing such a supplement to it, from the richness of his own invention.

I do not wonder however at no instrument pleasing Mr. Levret so well as his own. Nothing is more common among the instrumentarians, thank their disagreement about the make of their instruments. Some will have their forceps long, others short, some strait and flat, others curve: in short, there is no adapting the mechanism of it to their various fancies, so apt too as they are to change. Levret complains bitterly of the inability or injustice of the instrument-makers; but by what I believe of them, very unjustly. The gift of the fault is not in the instrument: it is in the use to which they are so often put of attempting impossibilities.

But now let us examine, what surely very competent judges have thought of this famous new forceps of Mr. Levret, which he calls *his* instrument.

When the book and instrument were presented the Royal Society at London, it appears by a quotation inserted by Mr. Levret himself, that his instrument was allowed to be ingenious enough, but that *"there was nothing extraordinary in it."*

Page the 10th of his preface, he has the candor to own, that he does not absolutely pretend that success will always attend its application, even in the cases he points out.

Page the 36th, and seq. of his observations, after having exploded the forceps, and other instruments of the authors who have preceded him; and after having described the alterations and corrections made in the English and French tire-têtes, he gives us indeed the better opinion of his, by a fair confession of the insufficiency of them all without exception, and even of his own: by which, however, it is plain, he can mean no more than that, imperfect as they are, they all are still preferable to the hands alone; but the question of this superiority is as constantly as it is shamelessly begged by him, and all his fraternity of instrumentarians.

Thus however he expresses himself as to his own instruments. "This instrument is actually, to all appearance, now at the very utmost degree of perfection, to which it is possible for it to arrive, without however having all the perfection that might be wished, for the most expert practitioners in the use of it, agree in the opinion.

"First, of the difficulty of its introduction in certain cases.

"Secondly, of its stubbornness as to the crossing of the blades.

"Thirdly, of its contributing to *tear* the *fourchette*, or *frænum labiorum*."

[Our author is very angry, that Boëhmer, who, in his critical objections, opposes those his own words to him, has not added the subsequent lines.]

"The correction I have made in this instrument (continues Levret) by means of the shifting axis, has rendered the difficulty of crossing the blades *less* considerable, and the two following reflexions may serve *greatly* to overcome the other two inconveniences."

But should it be granted to Levret, that the shifting axis somewhat lessens the difficulty of crossing the blades of this instrument, it would still remain too great an one, for all that correction. The reflexions he adds, for the overcoming the other two inconveniences, carry no conviction with them; and indeed he himself seems to think so, by his adding afterwards (p. 99.)

"To obviate this inconvenience of tearing the *fourchette*, or the perinæum, I caused to be made a *curve* forceps, as to any thing else not differing, in its dimensions, from the first. I took the idea of it, from the curve pinchers used in the operations of lithotomy. It will be easier to conceive, than for me to describe the advantage it must gain by it. That was not however the only end I proposed by it, as all the good practitioners at present agree on the *small* efficacy of the common forceps, in the case of a head struck in the passage when the face is turned upwards."

It is in consequence of this opinion that Levret, in the sequel to his observations, p. 301, tells us.

"I could (says he) answer Mr. Boëhmer, that all the most eminent men-midwives are convinced, that when the child presents with the face upwards, or turned forwards, that is to say, towards the os pubis, and that in this position, the head sticks, the forceps commonly used can be of *no* service: I do not (adds he) even except the one I have had made with a shifting axis. The defectiveness of these instruments, in these particular cases, sufficiently proves, I should think on one hand, that the English forceps is not so good as Mr. Boëhmer seems to believe; and on the other, I presume, he will be convinced, that I am not more servilely attached to my own productions, than those of others."

184

This insufficiency then of the common forceps has given rise to the curve forceps of our author. Here follows what he further adds to what I have above (p. 427) quoted from page 99 of his work.

"The form I have given to my forceps, renders it then very useful, since, by means of the curve, it lays holds of the head with all the efficaciousness that can be found in the use of the common forceps, employed on the most advantageous position that the head can be imagined ... Notwithstanding all the corrections made in the English and French forceps (continues the other practitioners) if my instrument is compared to all the other forceps it will appear;

"First, that it has none of their faults.

"Secondly, that it is very feasible with it to extract the head of a child separated from the body and remaining in the uterus. This is so possible, that all those who have seen my instrument, are unanimously of opinion, that no other forceps can do as much.

"Thirdly, with my instrument it appears to me possible to assist powerfully the getting out the head of a child that shall have remained in the uterus, the body being intirely come out, but of which a part is still in the vagina.

"Fourthly, my instrument has this in common with the ordinary forceps, that it can extract a child by the head, when this part shall be stuck in the passage."

It may well be said here, that Mr. Levret attributes such excellent qualities, and marvellous properties, to that same new forceps of his, as ought to immortalize his memory, and render his forceps universal over the whole earth,—if they were but proved. Ay! there lies the difficulty. Messieurs Rathlaw, Boëhmer, Jinckius, and the most notable practitioners in England, do not believe a syllable of the matter. Even Dr. Smellie, though I think he approves the crooked part of the forceps, speaks slightly enough of it, and has even dared to falsify the inventor's assertion of the ne-plus-ultra of it, by altering the form, as he tells us, p. 370. "in a manner that renders it more simple, more convenient, and lets expensive." Mr. Levret cannot then expect we shall take these advantages for granted upon his own bare assertion, in the blind enthusiasm he manifests for this rare production of his genius. I do not so much as believe, that he was even himself, at times, clearly persuaded of its excellence. At least he, in several places, appears to contradict himself. As it is then greatly of use to show into what a maze of errors these are capable of falling, who neglecting the guidance of judgment in the road of truth, wander into the wilds of imagination, I shall just point out here some of Levret's, at least, to me, seeming inconsistencies with himself, but especially with plain reason and common-sense. The reader will find the notice I take of them far from digressive, serving as they do even for connexion, as well as inforcement of my arguments.

Mr. Levret, p. 161, concludes the first part of his observation thus.

"Nota, some very intelligent persons have been pleased to charge me with an opinion, which I have never had as to CURVE FORCEPS: they think, that I believe it capable of going into the uterus in search of the child's head when it is not ingaged in the orifice: and yet I do not advise the use of it, unless in those cases where the other (the common forceps) is employed, over which it has essential advantages."

Here the reader will please to observe, that all the wonders, just before quoted from himself, are reduced only to the cases in which it may be advantageously substituted to the common forceps. This, by the by, is reducing it to less than nothing. But how is this consistent with those same marvellous excellencies he displayed to us a little before, to wit? *It is very feasible with it to extract the head of a child separate from the body, and remaining in the uterus."*—And again, *"with my instrument it appears to me possible, to assist powerfully the getting out the head of a child that shall have remained in the uterus, the body being entirely come out, but of which a part is still in the vagina."*

Now these two cases clearly imply, that Mr. Levret's curve forceps is capable of going into the uterus in search of the child's head, even when it is not engaged in the orifice: for here the case meant, is either that of a head remaining detachedly in the uterus, after having been severed or torn away from its body: or of a head not separated, but remaining in the uterus after the body shall have come out, and part of it is still in the vagina.

If therefore Mr. Levret's forceps had the advantage over the common forceps, confessedly insignificant in these cases, of being able to lay hold of these heads, he might be somewhat in the right to exalt it as he has done. But at present he must be wrong, which ever side he takes. The dilemma is self-evident. He is in the wrong to deny what he had certainly said. He is in the wrong to complain of being taxed with an opinion, which his own allegations prove he had entertained. I therefore refer Mr. Levret from himself to himself. If he did not believe, that his curve forceps had over all the rest the properties he sets forth, why has he so confidently affirmed them? and after affirming them, why would he hinder us from thinking that he believed what he affirmed?

I am here to observe, that if I have made use of the terms of "a head not *separated but remaining in the uterus after the body shall have come out, and part of it is still in the vagina*," it is purely because I would not change any thing in the expression of this celebrated instrumentarian. It is this exactness of quotation, that has made me conform myself to his manner of speaking, in my answer upon this difficulty. Otherwise, I own, I do not apprehend the propriety to his description of the case. It surprized me too the more, in so intelligent a writer as Mr. Levret, that he should represent to us a body come out of the uterus, and yet remaining in the vagina; as if, on such an occasion, the vagina could be distinguished from the orifice of the uterus. It is even stranger to me yet in Mr. Levret, for that he himself, in a note, p. 106, of his observations (by me before quoted) expressly says, that "when you are for using this forceps, it is absolutely necessary that the orifice of the uterus should be, as it were, totally erased or defaced;" so that the vagina and orifice should be laid into one. (See p. 180)

Here follows a much more material contradiction, rather however to common sense than to Levret himself, to which I intreat the reader's particular attention.

Observations, part the 2d, p. 160. Levret gives us the following preliminary general precept.

"There is, says he, a general precept by which it is established, that a surgeon ought never to thrust instruments into deep places, without guiding or conducting them with the hand, or with the extremity of the fingers of that hand that does not hold the instrument."

It is then to this general axiom strongly dictated by reason, and surely in no case more obviously so, than where the exquisitely tender texture of the uterus protests against committing its safety from the cruelest injuries, to the necessarily blind random agency of an iron and steel instrument, so palpably ungovernable in so remote, intricate, and slippery a place by even the most skilful hand[40]; it is, I say, in exception to this so salutary general precept, that Mr. Levret will have it that there are exceptions, and in favor of what, do you think, not surely of the poor woman who, is to be the subject, or rather the victim of the experiment, but of—his most egregiously silly CURVE FORCEPS! Yes; it is by way of trying practices with the same instrument, that the patient is liable to be *spread out*, in that delicate attitude which I have above, (p. 237) described from Levret, to the perusal of whom, for a thorough conviction of the perfect insignificance of that instrument, or indeed of any of that sort, I would recommend even the most sanguine in favor of instruments, if they would but grant, to their own reason, its just prerogative of a previous suspence of prejudice.

In these cases, however, for the which being exceptions to that excellent general rule, Levret contends; and, to do him justice, contends so auckwardly, that he rather provokes pity than indignation, at his endeavouring to establish even so pernicious an error; let the reader consider within himself the part into which this forceps is to be thus blindly thrust, at the risque of so many almost inevitable dangers. And for what?—In those cases it is either possible or not possible to introduce the fingers. Where they absolutely cannot be insinuated, the introduction of those instruments is in all human probability big with the worst of mischiefs, where neither hand nor fingers can controul the effects of the iron or steel: which, consequently, endanger more than they can help, and are therefore not to be used. But if the hand or the fingers can be insinuated, the hand or the fingers well conducted will do the work without the help of instruments, which in this second supposition become also useless.

---

[40] If any one doubts of this, he, in order to settle his opinion, needs but to peruse the instructions given by Levret, and other instrumentarians, for the use especially of the forceps. He will find such obscurity, such intrepidity of practices upon flesh not their own, as would make one shudder. They very cautions against *looking in* a part of the uterus between the blades of the instrument, prove the existence of a danger no caution can scarce answer for its being able to avoid. What do you think of young or unskilful practitioners thrusting up instruments at RANDOM into such a place? yet Dr. Smellie, p. 288, expressly tells you, there is a case in which "*The forceps* MUST *be introduced at random.*" This however may give the practitioner boldness, that whatever is his fault, the poor woman it is that is sure to suffer for it, and how cruelly!

This brings me to this case particularly, the title of which is prefixed to this section, that of a head stuck in the passage, which the gentlemen-midwives may perhaps second Levret, in maintaining to be an exception to that admirable axiom above quoted, and maintain it purely, in evasion of the conclusion against their miserable instruments, which I aver need never be resorted to, nor never are, but for want of sufficient skill in the manual function to terminate such labors without them.

I answer then to these instrumentarians, that an instrument, even, no more dangerous than a probe, would in so tender a place as I am treating of, not perhaps be quite enough exempt from a possibility of doing mischief, to deserve an exception: but as to those instruments, which are so palpably likely to hurt both mother and child, to injure, in short, or even to destroy both the mould and the cast, they are all of them within the case of exception, or rather exclusion. It is then, in knowing what to do, and in the faculty of operating with the hand according to that knowledge, that the art of midwifery principally consists. If instruments are deemed ingenious, the doing without them is surely not less so.

Now as to the case proposed in this section, that of a child's head stuck in the passage, I aver, that it is not absolutely impossible to terminate this delivery by the hand.

I am even ready to demonstrate this before any competent judges. I speak by experience. I have hitherto executed with all desirable success this operation without any aid but that of the hand, with a little patience and proper assiduity. I have many and many a time seen it practiced at the Hôtel Dieu, and elsewhere. I never in my whole course of practice saw sufficient reason for attempting so hazardous an extraction, as that which is executed by means of a tire-tête. Why then those needless terrors, those superfluous tortures with instruments, to women already in too much pain and anguish? care enough could not to be taken to spare those of the weaker-nerved sex in that condition such horrors, the very idea of which, to say no more, is enough to put them into imminent peril of their lives. All the forceps, and the rest of the chirurgical apparatus, especially the more complex instruments, very justly frighten the women, and their friends and assistents for them. Their introduction requires at once a painful, a shocking, and a needless divarication. The patients are put into attitudes capable of making them die with apprehension, if not with shame, from that native modesty of theirs, which, in these cases, may however be pronounced rather a wife instinct than a virtue.

How much preferable is the true midwife's practice, who will have oftenest prevented, by her knowledge and skill, this very situation! That is to say, if she has been called in time. She knows how to predispose the passages, and by gentle reductions to restore Nature to her right road, where she has been through mis-practice driven out of it, or through negligence suffered to deviate from it, or not preventively watched.

I have never but seen, with respect to the uterus in this case, that it was possible to insinuate first one finger, then another, and little by little the whole hand, not indeed a hard hand, as big as a shoulder of mutton, the hand of some lusty he-midwife, but of a midwife, such as it is commonly seen.

When Nature does not proceed as could be wished in her labor-pains, the point is then to husband well the strength of the patient, to restore it where it fails, by giving her good broths and corroboratives, that do not heat, or cooling things, where heating ones have been injudiciously administered. She is then to lie as composed and tranquil as possible; to be cherished, comforted, inheartened. There is, humanly speaking, no fear but her strength will return; her pains must not be irritated, nor herself harassed with ineffectual interference. Nature will come to herself again: the situation will, by her benign energy, change for the better, and become favorable enough, for the midwife to be able to assist her in the due time with a manual operation, that will terminate happily her delivery. It is at least, with this success, that I have delivered many, who, by the unskilfulness of those who had attended them, at the beginning of their pains, had been reduced to a deplorable condition, by their labor lingering some for upwards to six days.

In short, it is extremely rare that this case of a head stuck in the passage ever happens, unless under the hands of unskilful practitioners, or of over-dilatory or neglectful midwives, who will not have duly attended to the prognostics of this event; who will not have watched and taken the benefit of the favorable critical moment; who give the head time to engage itself, or get fast jammed, for want of their removing the impediments to Nature's doing the rest, or when help has been called or come too late. It may also be owing to those who hasten too much, who precipitate the women's labor by forcing draughts, that heat, burn them up, exhaust their strength, and prematurate the coming on of the labor-pains. Some practitioners fatigue them, with making them walk, or keep them up too much.

But when the membranes are not too soon pierced and the waters let out, when the pains are not provoked, when time is given to Nature to form to herself a passage, not omitting the precautions I have summarily intimated; when due care is taken to procure all possible ease of body and mind to the patient; who may vary her posture, sometimes lying along, sometimes sitting up, or well supported when she walks: little by little the head will frank itself a passage with the weight of the body acting by an innate energy, and with a little due assistance of the midwife's art: and with this practical advertence, that, in these arduous cases, much may be safely left to Nature, but not every thing. There are times in which she cannot bear neglect, but there are none in which she can bear extreme violence.

Here the reader will not expect I should in a treatise, purely calculated to expose the abuses of midwifery, attempt to particularize either all the contingent cases, or all the modes of operation in them. That would require a work a-part. I shall only then, to the four principal cases, in which instruments are so falsely supposed necessary, add a summary account of that of a *pendulous belly*, which is not without its difficulty.

As to a PENDULOUS BELLY, madam Justine, midwife to the Electress of Brandenbourg, remarks, in her Treatise of the Art, that she knows, by experience, that some children turn upon their heads with their feet upwards, in women who have a large and prominent abdomen; because, says she, they are pitched too much into the fore-part of the belly, that is become pendulous. But she does not explain the consequence of this situation, which however does not fail of causing a severe and troublesome labor; in that the uterus being fallen into the capacity of the hypogastrium, and the child being got above the os pubis, there it sticks, and the labor-pains are ineffectual, if proper assistance is not given to Nature.

The practice which my success on experience encourages me to propose is, to have the patient lye on her back, the belly to be braced upwards with a large linnen-fold or roller, to reduce the uterus and fœtus to its better position in the capacity of the pelvis; but if, notwithstanding that help, the head of the child continues to rest on the os pubis, the finger must be insinuated between

191

those bones and the head, in order to make, it, little by little, retrograde into the pelvis towards the coccyx.

In every case then that can be imagined, so far as my own experience and observation have reached, I am authorized to aver, that the gentleness of the manual assistance to women is at once more agreeable to Nature, and more salutary than the violence of the instrumental practice; which not only conveys the idea, but the very reality of a butchery. While its being sheltered under the plausible pretext of tenderness and pious regard to the safety of the poor women and children, cannot but provoke the greater indignation, at seeing vile interest trifling thus wantonly with their lives, and add to the cruel outrages on the human person, the greatest of insults on the human understanding.

It cannot however have escaped observation, that while I am, with the utmost regard to truth, endeavouring to recommend the preference of the hands to instruments, there is nothing I mean so little, as that some deliveries may not be accomplished by instruments, and especially by that divine invention of the forceps. What I presume to exclaim against, is the needless torture to the mother, the needless increase of danger to which she and her child both are exposed, for the sake of that practice being tried upon them, with those instruments, when the bare hands would be so much more safe and effectual. I could myself, no doubt, in many cases, if I could be inhuman and wicked enough to dally with any thing so sacred as the health or life of a woman and child, in some measure, intrusted to me, give myself the learned air of delivering with a CURVE FORCEPS. But in the very same cases, though at the hazard of being called ignorant for my pains, I would always be sure to do it more cleverly, less dangerously, less hurtfully, with only my hands. So that, without straining any comparison, the forceps may deliver indeed, but how? Why just as a man may, if he chuses it, hobble round St. James' Park, on a pair of those *artificial legs*[41], called stilts, when one would imagine, that the mock-elevation from them could scarce atone for their uncouth totteringness, and that he might full as well deign to use his own *natural* legs.

---

[41] "The forceps may be introduced with great *ease* and *safety*, like a pair of *artificial hands*, by which the head is very *little* (if at all) *marked*, and the woman very *seldom tore*." Smell. p. 257.

In the slighter cases then, that is to say, in those cases, where it is a jest to doubt of the hands not being the preferable instrument, since they may be truly avered to be so even in the most difficult ones, instrumentarians commonly go to work, *only* (please to mind that *only*) with the forceps. So that it is *only* in those slighter cases, where, once more nothing is more certain than that no instrument is wanted at all, that they find matter of triumph over their predecessors in theory and practice, over common sense, and especially over humanity. And this is that amazing, that FORTUNATE IMPROVEMENT, the superhuman invention of the forceps, the philosopher's stone of the modern art of midwifery, found out by the male-practitioners. Yet, after all it plainly appears, that even themselves do not rely on it in the more difficult cases. They are then obligated to return to the *old* crotchet, or the like methods, which bad, very bad, and very inferior to the hands as they are, never however are supposed to be resorted to, without an appearance of extremities to afford some color, some plea of humanity to employ them, in a kind of dernier resort, to prevent a greater evil by a less one. Whereas, when the forceps is used, the cruelty of that torture it cannot but create, must be greatly aggravated by the consideration of its being perfectly needless. But in the case of using either crotchet or forceps, or indeed any instruments at all, the truth is, that besides the increase of danger and pain they bring, to the already too much afflicted patients, they defraud them of the more efficacious, less painful, and especially more safe help of the hands alone.

The instrumentarians all then agree on that insufficiency of this pretious forceps, which occasionally compels their recourse to the crotchet so detested even by themselves. Levret, for example, confesses this, p. 24, of the appendix to his observations.

"The crotchets (says he) are, generally speaking, instruments, the very sight of which shocks and terrifies: but notwithstanding the repugnance which all *good* men-midwives ought to have to the using of them, there are cases in which there is no doing without them."

Now in these cases, that of the monster with two heads[42], is not meant to be included, as Levret himself afterwards explains himself. If then there are

---

[42] In this case of a monster of two heads, which happens so rarely as that it might almost be reputed null or of no consideration, *once more*, it is neither a midwife's business, nor even of one

such cases as necessitate a recourse to crotchets, it will, I presume, be allowed me, that they can be no other than those which render the delivery the most laborious. What those cases are, I have, from after the instrumentarians themselves reduced to the four capital ones, I have above set forth, without reckoning the pendulous belly. At least I know of no other situations than those, that can produce the very severe labors, nor do I believe that the instrumentarians know any other, or they would tell us so. Now if, in the more difficult of those cases, there is no doing without the crotchet, what becomes of the prodigious merit of the forceps, so insignificant in cases of the greatest need, and so superfluous in those others, where there being no occasion at all for it, it must be the most inhuman wantonness to employ it?

Here can you be with too much insistence desired to observe the solemn banter, in such a matter of life and death too, of these kind, tender-hearted modern instrumentarians! they are so transported with stark love and compassion to the poor women and children, that they do not know what they are about; they fall into the most palpable contradictions, and would have even Hippocrates, and the antients, appear as so many bloody-minded Cannibals compared to them. Hippocrates, it seems, and the antients, according to the best of their apprehension, in points of midwifery, prescribed the crotchet, in no case however but where the child was certainly dead, which, by the by, is next to the not prescribing it at all, since the ascertainment of that death is scarce not impossible. So because they recommended this practice in the last necessity, the ingeniousness of the modern instrumentarians was "[43]stimulated to contrive some *gentler* method of bringing along the head"—without any necessity at all; that is to say, in the minor difficulties, for the crotchet of the old practice is, to this instant, even with them, left in possession of the greater ones. Thus was produced the forceps, that prodigiously bright refinement upon the dull antients, and goes on improving without end under the wife heads of our gentlemen-midwives. But if the modern Genius of arts and sciences has no better improvement than this to boast over Hippocrates and the antients, may the instinct of self-preservation defend mothers, and, in them, their children, from being the

the common men-practitioners of midwifery. Application should be instantly made to one of the best and ablest surgeons procurable for reasons too obvious to need specification.

[43] Smellie, p. 248.

trophy-posts of their victorious atchievements! may the midwives continue in their happy ignorance of their curious devices! may they ever preserve a due aversion from indeed all instruments whatever! for they are all needless and pernicious substitutes to the hands. May none of them, especially in any labors committed to their conduct, prove so criminally false to their sacred trust, as through negligence, or through an interested designing reliance upon instruments, to repair their failures or mis-practice, slacken their attention to their duty, or afford, by their defective performance, an excuse, though a fallacious one, for resorting to instruments, when skilful hands are incomparably more fit for a remedy or retrieval!

I cannot then too ardently wish, for the women not to be so cruel to themselves, and to their so naturally dear children within them, as inconsistently to suffer their aim at superior safety, to be the very snare that betrays them into the greater danger, and often worst of consequences, from those male-practitioners, to whom that aim drives them for recourse; while that examination they owe to so interesting a point would issue, or deserve to issue, in rescuing them from such a shameful subjection of body and spirit to a band of mercenaries, who palm themselves upon them, under cover of their crotchets, knives, scissors, spoons, pinchers, fillets, *terebra occulta*, *speculum matricis*, all which, and especially their *tire-têtes*, or *forceps*, whether Flemish, Dutch, Irish, French or English, bare or covered, long or short, strait or crooked, flat or rounding, windowed or not windowed, are totally useless, or rather worse than good for nothing, being never but dangerous, and often destructive.

Nature, if her expulsive efforts are but, in due time, and when requisite, gently and skilfully seconded by the hands alone, will do more, and with less pain than all the art of the instrumentarians, with their whole armory of deadly weapons. The original and best instrument, as well as the antientest, is the natural hand. As yet no human invention comes near it, much less excells it: and in that part it is that the women have incomparably and evidently the advantage over the men for the operations of midwifery, in which dexterity is ever so much more efficacious than downright strength.

And, indeed, let every requisite faculty for the assistance of lying-in women be well considered, and the resulting determination cannot but be, that in the common labors, where the men themselves are either simple by-standers or receivers of the child, or operate with the hand only, they are the very best of them, not comparable to a common midwife, and in those cases, in which they pretended the use of instruments necessary, hardly better than the worst one. So that, not less than justly speaking, they are not receivable, either as substitutes, or even as supplements to midwives.

The art of midwifery then, in its management by women, carries with it, in the recommendation of order, modesty, propriety, ease, diminution of pain and danger, all the marks of the providential care of Nature. It is imaged by the incubation of a brood-hen, assiduously watching over her genial heat. Whereas the function of this art, officiated by men, has ever something barbarously uncouth, indecent, mean, nauseous, shockingly unmanly and out of character: and, above all, of lame or imperfect in it. It strongly suggests the idea of the chicken-ovens in Egypt, kept by a particular set of people, who make a livelihood of the secret, which they, it seems, ingross of that curious art of hatching of eggs by a forced artificial heat: a practice, which, like the other refinements of dung-beds for the same purpose, or that of committing the rearing or education of the chickens to [44]"*cocks*, to *capons*, or to *artificial wooden mothers*," may found indeed vastly ingenious; but besides the numbers that perish the victims of those experiments, many of the productions of such methods of hatching are observed to be maimed, wanting a leg or a wing, or some way damaged or defective. The comparison breaks indeed in that, at least, the grown hens themselves escape damage, which is not often the case of mothers under those heteroclite beings the men-midwives; or, if they do escape, it is no thanks to those operators, but to the prevalence of Nature over their pragmatical intervention, so fit to disturb, thwart, or oppose her effects, and in every sense to deprive the unhappy women that trust them of her common benefit.

But while superior considerations of humanity so justly intercede for the mothers, while I strenuously contend for the preference to be, without hesitation, due to the mother over the child, especially in that dreadful dilemma, where one must be sacrificed to the safety of the other; supposing such a dreadful alternative ever to exist, which I much doubt, or at least, not to exist so often as it is rashly taken for granted, and even then, where the

---

[44] See Reaumur's art of hatching domestic fowls, &c.

effects do not always follow the resolution taken thereon, since, though the child is always certainly lost, the mother is far from always saved, when, by a judicious preventiveness in practice, neither of them might perhaps have been so much as in jeopardy; while, I say, I plead for the preferable attention to the mothers, I hope no mothers will think me the worse intentioned towards them, for giving the lives of their children the second place in my tender concern for the safety of both.

And surely never was a time, when children more required the intercession of humanity in their favor. Mothers can speak for themselves. But the poor infants, so often precluded, by violence, from the pity-moving faculty of their own cry, have nothing but the cry of Nature to plead for them. A cry, the listening to which is prevented by those vain imaginary terrors, inspired by designing Art in the service of Interest, through which Nature is seduced to act against herself, and deliver herself up to her greatest enemies.

In short, one would imagine, that all the rage of cruelty was unchained, and let loose against especially those tender innocents, born or unborn.

Among the poor, particularly as to those infants cast upon the publick charity, a barbarously premature ablactation, under a pretext so easily foreknown to be as false as it is fatal, of bringing them up by hand for cheapness-sake, has destroyed incredible numbers.

Among the rich, or those able enough to pay for the learned murder of their offspring, how many of their children, even before they have well got hold of life, in this, literally speaking as to them, iron age, encounter their death or wounds, stuck in the brain by a crotchet, or crushed by a forceps, to say nothing of their being now and then ingeniously strangled in the noose of a fillet!

And those horrors proceed unchecked and unexploded, and in what a nation? a nation, that values herself upon the distinction of profound thinking: a nation that, besides that interest she has in common with all other well-governed nations, to protect and promote population, stands, be it said, in that true spirit of justice, which as much disdains to pay a fulsome compliment, as good sense ever will to receive it, moreover eminently distinguished above them all, for producing a race of natives, one would think could hardly be too numerous, since they are the most remarkable in the known world for courage, for personal beauty, and for many other liberal gifts of Nature, among which surely not the least is, that inborn spirit of liberty, to which they owe the honorable acquisition of so many additional advantages.

Can it then be too strongly recommended to the women especially, at least, to examine whether their notion of superior safety under the hands of a man, in their lying-in, bears upon the solid foundation of Nature, or merely on the treacherously weak one of a delusive opinion? an opinion that owes its existence to fears cruelly played upon, and turned to account by designing Interest. If those then of them who are under the force of prejudice, or governed by habit, or by both at once, would, on a point that concerns themselves and children so nearly, assume liberty enough of mind to shake off the dangerous yoke, they would undoubtedly find it better and safer to listen to that salutary instinct of Nature so authorized by reason, which inspires them with that repugnance to submit themselves in the manner they must do that submit themselves to men-midwives, who have the impudence to call that repugnance a "*false modesty*:" as if that Modesty could not be a true one, a foolish one I am sure it could not be, that should murmur at being so cruelly sacrificed to such a bubble's bargain as it is, by those innocents, who, over-persuaded by a deceitful promise of more effectual aid, too often embrace a torturous and a shameful death, for which, to add ridicule to horror, they are expected to pay their executioners larger fees than to one of their own sex for a more decent, a more safe, and always a less painful delivery.

May the women then, for their own sakes, for the sake of their children, cease to be the dupes, sure as they are to be in some measure the victims of that scientific jargon, employed to throw its learned dust in their eyes, and to blind them to their danger or perdition! may they, in short, see through that cloud of hard words used by pedants, whose interest it is to impose themselves upon them: a cloud, which is oftener the cover-shame of ignorance, than the vehicle of true knowledge, and perhaps oftener yet the mask of mercenary quackery, than a proof of medical ability!

As to the writings of the men-midwives especially, I dare aver, that, though there may be here and there some very just theoretic notions, borrowed from able physicians and surgeons, nothing is more contemptible than most of their practical rules; what is tolerable in them being most probably got from midwives, but so disfigured with their own absurd sophistications, that I should heartily pity any woman, subjected to have her labor governed by such, as should have no better guidance than their ridiculous instructions.

Then it is that a sensible woman would, in defence of her own life, or of any life that she holds dear to her, in the case of needing the aid of midwifery, view with equal disdain, with equal horror, either the rough manly[45] he-midwife, that in the midst of his boisterous operation, in a mistimed barbarous attempt at waggery or wit, will ask a woman, in a hoarse voice, "if she has a mind to be rid of her burthen," or the pretty lady-like gentleman-midwife, that with a quaint formal air, and a gratious smirk, primming up his mouth, in a soft fluted tone, assures her, and lies all the while like a tooth-drawer, that his instruments will neither hurt nor mark herself nor child but a little, or perhaps not at all. (See p. 448.)

This last character, if less brutal than the other, is not perhaps the least dangerous, since the practice being at bottom the same, pregnant consequently with the same mischief, the gentleness of the insinuation gives the less warning, and paves the way for the admission of a handling not the

---

[45] If any of my readers imagine that I have, in my objection to the men-midwives, exaggerated matters, I intreat of them to consider the following quotation from a *male-practitioner*, from Daventer, who endeavoured, as much as Nature would allow him, to be a good midwife, however he fell short of it. These are his own words translated, from p. II. of the French quarto edition.

"Can any thing be more shocking to the mother, and to those about her, than to see a man in liquor, scarce knowing what he is about, divested of all compassion, of all sentiment of humanity, his hands *armed* with a *knife*, a *crotchet*, a *pair* of *pinchers*, or other *horrible* instruments, come to the ASSISTANCE of a woman in agonies, begin, for his first attestation of skill, by *wounding* the *mother*, then go on to *destroy* the *child*, bring it away piece-meal, with exquisite tortures to the woman, and, after all, grumble in the notion, that he could not be PAID enough for such a fine spot of work? had not such better at once take on to be *butchers* or *hangmen*, than treat thus the image of God, and render the profession odious?"

Have I any where said any thing STRONGER than this? Daventer, however, certainly did not mean by it to insinuate, that *all* men-midwives answered intirely this description; no, nor I neither. But leaving the brutality out of the question, the mischief and mercenariness of them all differ perhaps in no very considerable degree. Please to remark in the following quotation, the DOCTRINE and practice of that famous *man-midwife* Peu. "He determines himself, without much ceremony, to the *breaking* a child's *arm* or a *thigh*, when he *imagines* this *operation* will facilitate the delivery, and that, on the PRINCIPLE of is being *easy*, to repair such *damages* of *new-born* infants. For the same reason the luxation of a jaw-bone gives him no scruple." (Translator of Daventer's Preface.)

less rough for the smoothness of the address. But is there any such thing as polite murder? is mischief the less mischief for being perpetrated with an air of kindness? well considered it is but the more provoking. The male-practitioners then are not quite in the wrong, to presume as they do upon the weakness of the women's understanding, since they can so grossly pass upon them their needless cruelties, under so inconsistent and false a color as that of a tender compassion. Thus to all the rest of the shame to which they put them, they add that of so palpable an imposition in that flimsy cover of the mean interest, which is so probably the real motive at bottom of their taking up a function, to which they were never called by Nature, nor by any necessity, unless, perhaps, of their own.

In the mean time, the truth is, that, in vain, would the men, by way of sparing the women the terror of their masculine figure, upon those delicate occasions of officiating, and to appear the more natural in the business, aim at an occasional effemination of their dress, manner and air. They can never in essentials atone for their interested intrusion into an office, so clearly a female one, that, if but only as to the manual discharge of it, not even the qualifying them for the opera, would, perhaps, sufficiently emasculate them.

CONCLUSION OF THE SECOND AND LAST PART.

Here, confessing my just apprehensions of not having fulfilled the promise of my title-page; there will not, I hope, to that reproach of my deficient powers in the performance, be added the undeserved ones of vanity or injustice in the design or conduct of my feeble essay.

For as to vanity, or any presumption, on my part, of anything so weak, so unauthoritative as my representation, having any chance to remove the abuses, not however the less existent for that incapacity of mine to remove them, my knowledge of the world would alone defend me from so ridiculously wild a thought. I am but too well aware of the tenaciousness of especially false prejudice in most minds, where it has once gained entrance, and with whom prepossession is ever eleven points of the right. I have then purely had in view the discharge of that duty, incumbent on every member of human society, to oppose such errors as appear to be pernicious to the good of it. In that light I have beheld the growing practice of the instrumentarians, and in that sincere belief I have hazarded the publication of my sentiments, without surely pretending to any authority over the opinion of others. That I cheerfully leave to every one's reason, who is capable of reason. And to write for others than the rational, would be only labor deservedly lost.

As to injustice, I am, at least, clear of that of partiality to my own sex. I grant and lament as much as any one the incompetency of but too many of the midwives. The number of such cannot be too little. But then would the banishing them out of the practice be preferable to the having them better taught, especially since there is nothing but what is so much worse to put in their room, men and instruments? What occasion too for such a dangerous extremity? For as the deficiency is evident, so are the causes: which are not only the want of sufficient care in the training and education of women to this profession, but the actual discouragement, which must grow every day greater and greater, by the incroachments of the instrumentarians, whose plea for supplanting them will be consequently strengthened by that alarming scarcity of capable midwives, which themselves will have so much contributed to create. These being then the principal causes, and well known to be so, the remedies are not obscure, nor hard to attain.

A good education especially is of great importance, to accomplish what Nature has already gone so great a way in, by her giving in many respects to the women such a superior aptitude for the business. Capable midwives would much help to form good female pupils; and the lying-in hospitals especially might be made highly useful to desirable an end. But surely as to the practical part of midwifery in these hospitals, it ought not to be under the direction of men, whose interest it should be, only to form the women so deficiently, as that themselves might be the less unnecessary; to form them, in short, more for their own service, than for that of the public. That temptation being removed, the female-practitioners could not receive too respectfully from the surgeons lectures or instructions, any lights in anatomy relative to their theoretic proficiency. But to nothing should they be more constantly and effectually excited, than to perfect themselves in the manual operation; and indeed, in general, so to capacitate themselves for their function, as to prove and establish the perfect inutility of all instruments whatever. Nor will it be a difficult task for a woman to acquire a superiority in her hands to the most boasted of those unnatural substitutes. This is the true way of laudably disarming the instrumentarians, and of thereby depriving them of the only shadow of a pretence they have for supplanting the women, and invading the female province, of which invasion it is so probable, that not the cause they plead, but the pay they squint at, is the real motive.

As to the discouragement of proper women from applying themselves to the profession, it can only cease by the concurring of those, on whom the choice out of either sex occasionally depends, to restore things to their antient channel: and that will in course, for their own sakes, follow on their ceasing to be imposed upon by the false pretences of the men-practitioners. But this is a point upon which I am too much a party to be heard, though even as no more than an advocate, and much less as a judge. All I shall then presume to say is, that I very readily leave the decision of the question to Reason, that inward oracle in every one's breast; an oracle, which, in a cause so interesting to human Nature, can never return a false answer, where consulted by those who deserve to find the truth by sincerely seeking it; with a firm design to sacrifice to it the poor vanity of defending a prejudice, or any other interest of the passions. And surely there can hardly exist a point of more capital importance to Society, than the determining, what however one would imagine not very difficult to determine, on which side in this profession of midwifery particularly, the superiority of auxiliary power may be expected, on that, where there is evidently a great deal of Nature, assisted with a little but a competency of Art, or on that, where what there is of Art is most barbarously abused, and without any Nature at all.

THE END.

www.ingramcontent.com/pod-product-compliance
Lightning Source LLC
Chambersburg PA
CBHW031851200326
41597CB00012B/359